MEDICAL
SCHOOL

MEDICAL SCHOOL

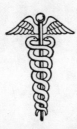

THE DRAMATIC TRUE STORY OF HOW FOUR YEARS
TURNED A CLASS OF RAW STUDENTS
INTO QUALIFIED PHYSICIANS

BY

DONALD DRAKE

RAWSON ASSOCIATES PUBLISHERS, INC.

NEW YORK

The names and other identifying characteristics
of all patients named in this book
have been changed in order to protect their privacy.

LIBRARY OF CONGRESS CATALOGING IN PUBLICATION DATA

DRAKE, DONALD
MEDICAL SCHOOL.

INCLUDES INDEX.
1. PENNSYLVANIA. UNIVERSITY. SCHOOL OF MEDICINE.
2. MEDICAL EDUCATION—UNITED STATES. I. TITLE.
R747.P492D72   1978   610'.7'1174811   78–54691
ISBN 0-89256-065-7

Published simultaneously in Canada by McClelland and Stewart, Ltd.
Manufactured in the United States of America
by Fairfield Graphics, Fairfield, Pennsylvania

Designed by Helen Barrow
First Edition

Dedicated to the two different drummers in my life
who started me along a path that few other people
seemed to be traveling—
My saintly mother, Gloria, and my charming father, Al.
And to my daughter, Valerie,
who I hope will hear the same beat.

ACKNOWLEDGMENTS

_____

I would like to thank many people in several different areas for making this book possible. First, since this book is based upon a four-year-long series that appeared in the Philadelphia Inquirer, *I would like to thank the executive editor, Gene Roberts, for establishing such a creative milieu in his newspaper that a demanding series of this type could be done. I would also like to thank David Boldt, the first editor I ever mentioned the idea to, for his surprising encouragement with the comment: "Four-year-long series! Sounds like a hell of an idea." And I would like to thank John Carroll, the metropolitan editor, who accepted the fact that his medical staff, which was me, would be neglecting daily stories in favor of this effort. And finally, Max King, a friend and an editor who worked with me on many of the stories.*

Next I would like to thank some people over at the University of Pennsylvania School of Medicine. I realize it was not easy for conservative academicians in medicine to accept the fact that a writer would be poking around their hospitals for four years. I would like to thank Edward J. Stemmler for taking the chance, even though there were many who advised him against it. I would also like to thank Mrs. Carol MacLaren, assistant dean for student affairs, who helped me gather statistical data and other tedious information without ever groaning in my presence, and Mrs. Katheryne Gantz, director of medical school admissions, who was equally helpful and friendly.

Finally I would like to thank all of the medical students who subjected themselves to interviews and having me follow them around in the hospitals when they were having enough trouble just trying to do their stuff in the alien world of medicine. It was not easy for them, especially because of the pressures from classmates, who were jealous or annoyed that a writer should be in their holy sanctum. Particularly I would like to thank:

Rikki Lights for her creativity, energy, spirit, rebellious nature, and for finding a guy like Ron Gilliam, who I would also like to thank.

Mark Reber for his sensitivity, empathy, and his delightful wife, Karen.

Steve Levine for his cogent perceptions and angry honesty.

Jim Nestor for his worldly wisdom, equanimity, and for his wife, Becky, whom he calls one of the "peak experiences of my life."

Matt Lotysh for his street smarts and unerring accuracy in assessing people's needs and expectations.

Randy Wiest for his quiet strength and determination to do his thing and not be co-opted by the system.

Marge Shamonsky for her courage to question and not be intimidated by those louder than she.

And finally, Helene Silverblatt, one of the most gentle, feeling, and aware people I have ever met, someone who will undoubtedly bring to the field of psychiatry, which she is entering, a quality it sorely needs.

I cannot help but think that medicine in this country will be improved because these people are becoming a part of it.

MEDICAL
SCHOOL

1

The one hundred letters were stacked in a small pile in the outgoing box of the admissions office. They didn't look very important. They were written on the inexpensive yellow letterhead of the University of Pennsylvania School of Medicine. They were mechanically produced to give the impression of being personally typed. And despite the great effort that went into deciding who should get them, no one in the office was particularly concerned about the letters any longer, at least not enough to hand-carry them to the mail room. Instead the one hundred letters languished in the outgoing box, waiting for an indifferent messenger to whisk them into his basket and start them on their way across the nation.

It was December 10, the day the school of medicine traditionally mailed the first batch of acceptance letters to eager pre-med students, telling them that they were among the lucky ones chosen to study medicine at Penn. They were being accepted as first-year students who would begin studies next September as members of the class of '78. Considering how important the letters were to the recipients, it was incongruous how casually they were treated.

Excluding addresses and names, the letter was seventy-two words long and said quite simply that the applicant had been accepted. That's what the words said, but the letter meant a lot more.

For one thing, it meant that the student had beaten the odds and gotten into an American medical school. Only one out of 2.8 applicants are accepted. And at a school like Penn—one of the most outstanding in the nation—the odds are much greater. For this particular first-year class, 4,124 persons had applied. Only 160 would get in.

Since few students who finally enter medical school drop out and fewer still are failed, the letter of acceptance is a virtual guarantee that the student will become a physician. This means that he will enter the most prestigious and highest-paid profession, one that will enable him to earn a good living in practically any part of the world he wants. Though many people, especially in the United States, will attack the profession, the individual practitioner will be treated as someone special wherever he goes

—a modern-day priest who has special secrets about life, death, and pain.

Though it's hard to measure how much the prestige and mobility is worth, the financial gains can be estimated. A typical physician in the United States makes $55,000 a year, almost double the average for most other professions, or about $2 million over a thirty-five-year professional career.

Looked at in this way, each of the one hundred letters being mailed this day almost guaranteed the recipient $1 million in extra income, prestige of immeasurable value, and an opportunity to live comfortably most anywhere in the world.

□ □ □

Among the 4,124 applicants waiting to hear from Penn was Matthew Lotysh, a personable, twenty-six-year-old former abalone diver, insurance salesman, and graduate student in physiology. Even though Matt wasn't a tall man, he looked powerful because of his big chest and arms, made muscular by the swimming and an athletic life. Matt spoke with a soft intensity and had a way of impressing people with his sincerity and self-awareness, characteristics that had aided him immeasurably as a salesman.

Matt had wanted to be a physician ever since he was a sixteen-year-old, when he was almost killed by the incompetence of one doctor, who repeatedly misdiagnosed Matt's belly pain as a muscle strain, and saved by the brilliance of another doctor who was hastily summoned after Matt's appendix finally ruptured.

Over the next ten years, Matt's boyish fantasy of emulating the surgeon who saved him turned into the unbreakable resolve of a compulsive young adult who wanted nothing else in life but to become a surgeon.

But now, as the time finally approached for Matt to go to medical school, his prospects did not look good. Matt had flunked out of his first year at college, and when he came back for a second try was able to achieve a grade point average (GPA) of only 2.2, which is a low C.

Matt's college advisers tried to discourage him from his long-held goal because, they said, the competition was too great for him to succeed. Practically all students who get into medical school have at least a B average. In fact 39 percent of the successful applicants the year before had a 3.6 GPA, which is an A or only four tenths of a point short of a perfect score of 4.

But Matt persisted in his determination and sent applications to nineteen medical schools. Within three weeks he had been rejected by every school. He didn't even get an interview. So he waited a year and tried again, this time sending out eleven letters. Eight schools immediately rejected him.

So here he was waiting for the last couple of letters to trickle in, putting all his hopes on the University of Pennsylvania because this was the only school at which he had managed to get an interview.

Matt had left the Penn interviews feeling high. He knew they had gone well. He was sure that they couldn't refuse him. The faculty people he talked to didn't seem at all concerned about his low marks. They were impressed by the research he was doing as a graduate student at the University of California in Davis. They were very interested in how he had started his own business diving for abalone.

These were the hopeful thoughts going through Matt's head as he flew west to wait for Penn's decision. But the days turned into weeks and still he heard nothing. The black feelings started to come. Could he have misjudged his reception at Penn? Was he doomed by those low undergraduate grades? Were his advisers right after all? If he failed again this year, would it serve any purpose to try the schools again next year?

Once back home Matt threw himself into his studies at Davis, where he was working in the dog lab on heart physiology. Compulsive about this work, he'd operate on a half-dozen dogs a day and go to the lab six or seven days a week. He was fascinated by the work. But always in the back of his mind was the ache of wanting to become a physician, a cardiovascular surgeon who operated on human beings instead of animals.

The ache came back every afternoon when he returned home from the laboratory and opened his mailbox. Checking the mail had become a ritual of great importance, like looking in the newspaper for lottery numbers. About three weeks after the Penn interviews, Matt opened the mailbox and found the yellow letterhead of the University of Pennsylvania Medical Center. It was lying in the box with a telephone bill and an advertising circular from *Time* magazine. Matt picked up the letter without opening it.

My God, it's not a rejection, Matt thought. Unlike all the rejections he had received, this envelope was much thicker. Only a single sheet was needed to reject an applicant. Acceptances required loan applications for study and instructions on what had to be done now. Matt still didn't open the letter. It was too important. He had counted on this moment too long, considered it, fantasized about what it would be like.

Walking the two hundred feet to his house, Matt went up to his apartment and got a can of beer from the refrigerator. Taking a drink of beer, Matt opened the phone bill and reviewed the charges. Then he scanned the magazine advertisement circular. Finally he opened the envelope from the University of Pennsylvania. The letter was written with little eloquence, but Matt read the words again and again and again. Signed by Dr. Richard H. Schwarz, chairman of the admissions committee, the letter read:

"It gives me great pleasure to extend to you a cordial invitation to become a member of our entering class for September, 1974.

"The conditions upon which this offer is based, and instructions with regard to the procedure to be followed, will be found in the enclosed statement. Please review these carefully.

"We look forward to your answer, and we hope that you will be with us in the fall."

□ □ □

There's no single thing an undergraduate student can do to guarantee that he or she will get into medical school. Good undergraduate marks are important, but they're not everything, since schools like Penn have rejected many students with a GPA of 4. The academically perfect student almost invariably will get an interview, but the admissions committee may then turn him down because his interests don't appear broad enough or his personality fails to impress the interviewers.

The school is looking for bright students who have demonstrated initiative and a lot of energy, not simply a dedication to medical science. Since so many applicants have high grades, this factor alone is not sufficient to pick the most able. Because of this, the selection process tends to be somewhat subjective and arbitrary in choosing all but the most gifted of the applicants. The applicant's ability to relate to his interviewers and reveal the qualities the interviewer can identify with becomes an important factor in the final phase of the selection procedure.

Most applicants don't even get a chance to put their personalities up for review. At Penn half the applicants are rejected without interviews by Mrs. Kathryn Gantz, the director of admissions. A friendly woman with graying hair, Mrs. Gantz relates to the students like a concerned but shrewd grandmother. Mrs. Gantz' primary job at this stage of the process is to check out questionable applicants, looking for qualities that merit special consideration. Such was the case with Matt, who, despite his low marks, demonstrated unusual energy and initiative by working his way through college as an abalone diver and insurance salesman and by doing fairly sophisticated research in heart physiology.

About a thousand of the applications that pass through Mrs. Gantz' original screening are rejected by a seven-member faculty committee, leaving only about eight hundred applicants for interviews. These students are invited to Philadelphia on Saturdays from October through February. Each is interviewed for a half hour by a faculty member and then for another half hour by a medical student.

Then at noon all of the interviewers meet and vote on who should be accepted from that day's pool of interviewees. So at Penn, at least, if a student makes it through to the interview, he has about a 25 percent chance of being offered a place in the upcoming first-year class.

The class of '78, which the committee and Mrs. Gantz was putting together, would have 22 minority students, all black, and 48 women out of the total of 160, the largest numbers of minority students and women in the school's history.

Despite the diversity, however, the typical medical student in this class, as well as in the first-year classes of most of the other 113 medical schools in the country, would be a white male from a middle-class background—probably the son of a physician—who was always at the top of his class from kindergarten through college. He would tend to be a compulsive person who never put off to tomorrow what he could do today. And most important, he would have a sense of mastery over his own destiny. He would decide precisely what to do with his time and life rather than leaving such things to chance or the whims of other people. Such a student would be Randy Wiest.

□ □ □

At twenty-one, Randy was a good-looking youth with a strong chin and athletic body. He spoke with the mild-mannered assurance of someone accustomed to achieving his goals.

Unlike Matt, Randy knew that he would get into medical school. He was a top student with a 3.9 GPA, had a diverse background of extracurricular activities, and was very interested in the outdoors and camping.

He had everything going for him. But for a long time Randy wasn't sure he wanted to become a physician. Medicine seemed too demanding a life for him to be happy with. He knew because his father was a physician.

Randy was one of the new generation of Americans, far removed from the economic and personal insecurities engendered by the Great Depression and military drafts and war. Raised in a comfortable if not affluent home, Randy had the freedom of mind to believe that there were more important things than the prestige of being a professional or the economic security that it brought.

Randy loved the outdoors and the leisure of relating to people and things in his environment. His father had always been so busy, away from the home, taking care of other people's problems. He had little leisure for anything.

But Randy also saw in his father's life the good things that medicine offered, the satisfaction of helping and being important to many people who turned to him for help. Also Randy realized that the profession could offer him the geographical freedom of working almost anywhere with a variety of practices to choose from. The thought of being a rural family physician was a delightful one to Randy. It was this thought that pushed Randy over the line and made him decide to become a physician.

Randy sent out applications to ten medical schools, concentrating on the seven schools in his home state of Pennsylvania. He knew this would give him an advantage over the out-of-state applicants. Interviews were offered without hesitation, and in no time Randy had been accepted by six schools, including the Hershey Medical Center, where his father was on the faculty, and the University of Pennsylvania.

The yellow envelope from Penn happened to arrive while Randy was home visiting from Penn State, where he was an undergraduate. Opening the letter in the kitchen, Randy read the contents to his parents.

For most of the applicants, receiving the seventy-two-word letter was a cause for celebration. But for Randy, it created a dilemma. He had already been accepted to five other schools and was leaning toward going to Hershey. Hershey was the only one of the Pennsylvania schools that was in the country, and he would have chosen it without reservation except that he didn't want to go to a school where his father was on the faculty.

Being the most prestigious school in the state and one of the most prestigious in the nation, Penn was a very appealing opportunity. But Randy didn't want to live in a city. And he wasn't happy about the impersonal atmosphere at Penn or the Penn people who had interviewed him.

The faculty interviewer had asked him which he was more interested in, research or teaching, as though these were the only options and small group practices didn't exist. And when Randy told the student interviewer that he wanted to become a rural practitioner, the student scoffed at him, saying that the new specialty of family practice was only a fad.

Sitting around the kitchen table with the open Penn letter before them, Randy and his father discussed the relative merits of the many opportunities. Randy's father had gone to Penn. He suggested that Randy had had a bad single experience in Philadelphia. They decided to go back to Philadelphia together and inspect the campus and talk to the students and faculty.

Unlike the Hershey Medical Center, a new medical school plunked down in the middle of the farmlands of central Pennsylvania, the University of Pennsylvania sits on the corner of a black ghetto in west Philadelphia. The nearest body of water is the polluted Schuylkill River, so contaminated at times by oil and gasoline that the fumes harass pedestrians on the many bridges crossing it. The only grass is on ball fields or in small plots. And the few trees are hemmed in by concrete and buildings.

Randy was oppressively aware of these things when he went back to Philadelphia with his father. But on this trip his father showed him some of the positive things about Penn.

Started in 1765 as the first medical school in the Americas, Penn was filled with a sense of medical history and tradition that couldn't help but impress the young people about to enter the profession. The ancient, classical-style medical college building was hidden away from the bustle of city traffic behind the turreted undergraduate dormitories. And Hamilton Walk, the walkway that connected the medical school to the University of Pennsylvania Hospital, was beautiful, shaded by leafy trees that muffled sounds and provided a sense of serenity. If Randy decided on

Penn, he'd spend almost all of his first year on Hamilton Walk or in the buildings along it.

Randy found the students on this visit much friendlier than the one who had interviewed him several weeks earlier. They told him that Penn had a low-pressure atmosphere. There were no numerical grades—only pass, fail, or honors. Students could elect almost half their courses rather than being pinned down by a rigid set of requirements. And most impressive of all, students saw patients during the first weeks of classes, unlike at other schools where there was no patient contact until the third year.

Randy thought about these things as he drove home with his father. The car sped west on the Pennsylvania Turnpike toward the green undulating farmlands of central Pennsylvania. It felt good to leave the gray and noise of the city behind. The city would be a cold, hard place to live in, Randy thought, staring pensively out of the car window. But there would be weekends and vacations. Randy hadn't expressed it yet, but there was no doubt in his mind now. He would go to Penn.

In the coming years, Randy would discover that his concern about the impersonal and competitive urban world he was about to enter had been well founded. He would learn that academic excellence in medicine wasn't achieved without sacrificing many qualities that Randy valued. And many times Randy would ask himself if he had made the right choice in going to Penn and deciding to become a physician.

□ □ □

Medical education in this country has undergone radical changes since the nation's social consciousness was goaded by the hectic, protest years of the 1960s. Becoming disenchanted with esoteric science that had little immediate value to the average person and medical advances that were available to only a few, the public demanded changes.

The people wanted more physicians and a better medical delivery system that would reach the poor and rural peoples of the country, not just the affluent. Woven into these demands was the thread of an intensified social awareness that blacks and women were being discriminated against by business, the professions, and education. Nowhere was that discrimination more apparent than in the white, male-dominated medical profession.

In 1969 more than half the nation's population was female and 12 percent were black. But in that year only 9 percent of entering students were women and 4.8 percent were black.

Pressured by these long-ignored concerns and aided by new federal funds, the medical educators responded forcefully. By the early 1970s, as Randy and Matt were preparing to enter medical school, a new type of student was being trained and in much greater numbers than before. In only a decade the number of medical schools has increased from 89 to 117 in 1977. And in half that time the number of first-year students has jumped 35 percent from 11,300 in 1970 to 15,300 in 1975.

With emphasis now being placed on getting good care to everyone instead of esoteric care to just a few, the twenty-year-long trend toward specialization has started to reverse itself. Instead of picking surgery or the even more highly specialized fields, the socially conscious students of the 1970s are choosing primary care medicine. They want to become general pediatricians, obstetrician-gynecologists, or family practitioners, the modern equivalent of the old-time GP, only much more highly trained.

In many schools, such as Penn, the curriculums have been changed, giving students much more freedom to custom-make their own education and study the courses that interest them. Out of the 32 course units required for graduation, only 17.5 of them consist of required courses. So many of the courses are elective that a Penn student could graduate without ever having delivered a baby or splinted a broken bone.

The new curriculums, changes in social consciousness, and the increased numbers of physicians are destined to change the type of doctor who will practice medicine in coming years. Of all the things happening, however, nothing will have a bigger effect on the quality or style of that practice than the sharp increase in the number of women and minority students entering medical school.

Until the late 1960s, very few women and even fewer minority students would dare to think about entering the white-male bastion of American medicine. Even though the acceptance rate for women was higher than for men, very few women considered medicine as a career. It wasn't a socially accepted career for women, and this taboo persisted for decades. Just before the Second World War only 5.4 percent of applicants were women. By 1960 that percentage had increased only to 6.9.

But then came the civil rights movement and women's liberation. By 1971 the percentage of women applicants jumped to 12.8. And by 1974 it was 20.4 percent. Forty-eight of the students in Randy's and Matt's class would be women. That's 30 percent. And twenty-two would be minority students.

With so many in the class, the women and minority students would not, as those before them had, think of themselves as oddities or token concessions to a vague social conscience. They would constitute a significant proportion of their class. Blatant sexism or racism would no longer be encountered. But there would be problems.

These students would have difficulty finding suitable role models because so few of the faculty and so few of the house officers in the hospitals would be women or nonwhites. And these students would always be aware that everything they did as people and as professionals would be judged by their highly critical peers and superiors in the context of their race and sex. They would not be able easily to forget that they were representing their sex or race in a professional world that had yet to accept them as competent.

Some of the blacks would have trouble relating comfortably to the white middle-class male students who had been programed from birth to enter the profession. And the women would always have to wonder about how feminine they dare be in dress or manner so as not to provoke the ire of the males around them. To be too feminine would be to provoke patronizing male chauvinism; to be too masculine would be to lose their identity as women and provoke disrespect for themselves as people. The coming four years would be difficult ones for women and minority students. They would be particularly difficult for the seven students who were both women and black—students like Vernether (Rikki) Lights.

Rikki Lights had every reason to expect an acceptance letter from Penn. Her undergraduate college, Bryn Mawr, is a prestigious women's college, just a few miles from Penn and historically a dependable source of women medical students. Rikki's GPA of 3 was low by white standards, but higher than the average for successful black applicants. And the large amount of writing she had done as a promising playwright and poet couldn't help but impress the Penn admissions committee.

But Rikki was convinced that she had blown the interviews. The faculty member who interviewed her didn't seem impressed by her being a writer. And the student who interviewed her as part of the admission process was not a minority student, as promised, but a white, blue-eyed, blond-haired, middle-class male.

Such a person could not possibly understand who she was or where she was coming from as a black woman in America, or so Rikki was convinced.

Rikki could never, for long, forget her sex and race. Whenever she failed for inexplicable reasons or ran into obstacles other people escaped or found people threatening or rude or condescending, she would wonder how much of this was because she was a black or because she was a woman or because she was both.

Trying not to think about having failed the Penn interview, Rikki resigned herself to the inevitability of such injustice and took comfort from the fact that she had already been accepted to Harvard and Boston universities. To make either school, especially Harvard, was a considerable accomplishment for anyone, but Rikki wanted to stay in Philadelphia.

Coming from Sea Island, a poor black community off the coast of South Carolina, Rikki did not easily adjust to big city life. It had taken her almost all of the four years at Bryn Mawr to work her way into a world of musicians and artists, and now she was reluctant to leave this support system, even to go to Harvard. She didn't want to spend the next four years building up another network of friends in Boston.

It would be difficult enough entering this new and foreign world of medicine. The prospect was particularly frightening for someone like Rikki, the twenty-one-year-old daughter of a former Marine Corps cook. In her poor hometown, a doctor was an oddity, someone people traveled far to see and only when they were very sick. Teachers were the only professionals who lived on Sea Island. The only other professional role models were actors Rikki saw on television or in movies.

Still she wanted to become a physician because, like so many other gifted blacks, she felt this was the most effective way she could improve the lot of her people. She would always write poems and books and jazz operas about blacks, but this would be to satisfy an inner need and abstract goal. The deep satisfaction of helping someone she could see and touch and relate to as an individual would come from medicine.

Rikki had no illusions about how difficult her life would be as a medical student. Not only would she have to adjust to a profession in which there were few blacks or women, but she would also have to balance the competing demands of two lives going in different directions.

In the daytime Rikki would live in the conservative, reserved, intellectual world of white physicians. And at night she would groove in the vibrant, explosive, and emotional world of black musicians. Somehow Rikki would have to develop a breadth of emotion and intellect to encompass both cultures. Rikki was concerned about this, but she was prepared to do it and knew that she would succeed. She did not know, however, if she would relate well with the other students in the class.

But she was prepared for this difficulty also. She would spend all her energies in the daytime studying and learning medicine. For social support and emotional release, she would turn to her writing at night and her life in the subculture of artists. But this option was contingent upon getting into Penn.

Her fears of being rejected reached a climax when she opened her mailbox on the Bryn Mawr campus and saw the letter from Penn lying there.

This is it, she said to herself at the instant of recognition. *The time has come to start those moving plans.*

Rikki picked up the letter and immediately she knew. Her fingers told her. It was a thick letter like the ones from Harvard and Boston universities. She had been accepted by Penn. No need to leave Philadelphia. She could stay. She was going to Penn.

Rikki ripped open the envelope. The first five words told her that it was true. "It gives me great pleasure," the letter started. That was it. The rest of the letter was anticlimactic. No need to read further because those five words said it all. "It gives me great pleasure."

"I do thank you," Rikki said, talking to the letter. "And it gives me great pleasure to accept." And off she ran to find Ron, her boyfriend, was a jazz musician. She wanted to tell him the big news. She wouldn't have to leave after all.

☐ ☐ ☐

Do some medical school applicants have an advantage in the competition because of their sex, age, race, or socioeconomic status? Judging from the composition of medical school enrollments, it would seem that the odds are tilted heavily in favor of white middle-class males. But almost the reverse is true. The only reason there are more of them is because more of them apply.

The most promising applicant these days is a young Chicano woman who has high marks and a physician for a father. She is in the honors program in undergraduate school. Her major is either philosophy or interdisciplinary subjects. And she's not from a poor home. The family income is over $50,000 a year.

This, at least, is the composite picture of the perfect applicant as drawn from the statistical review of applicants made each year by the Association of American Medical Colleges (AAMC).

Though grades clearly may be the single most important factor, they are not the only thing, and even the best of marks can't guarantee an applicant a place in medical school. It is true that students with a perfect GPA of 4 are the most likely successful applicants. Eighty percent of the A students were accepted as compared to only 10 percent of applicants with GPAs below C or 1.99 or less. But still 20 percent of the A students were rejected.

Some of them failed because their college admission test scores weren't impressive. But even students with near perfect MCATs (Medical College Admissions Tests) in the 700s and perfect GPAs of 4 didn't always make it. In fact, 8 percent of the 105 academically perfect students in the 1975–76 applicant pool were rejected, for unspecified reasons.

If perfect grades don't mean everything, then what were the other important factors as revealed by the AAMC study?

AGE

New federal law may prohibit discrimination on the basis of age, but age is clearly a handicap when it comes to getting into medical school. Forty percent of applicants in their early twenties make it into medical school as compared to only 18 percent of those who are in their early thirties.

The chances for success decline with advancing years, going from a 56 percent acceptance rate for those under twenty-one to 8 percent for those over thirty-seven.

SEX

Women have a slightly better chance of succeeding than men. Thirty-eight percent of the women who applied in 1975 were accepted as compared to only 35.7 percent of the men. Unlike minority group applicants, women are not given an advantage in the competition. It's just that their grades are slightly higher on the average, and other factors, such as personal warmth, tend to impress admission committees more.

Ironically, partly because of the women's movement, the percentage of women *applicants* accepted has actually declined in recent years, going from 45 percent in 1971 to the current 38 percent. That's because the change in social mores has encouraged more women, including academically less gifted ones, to seek medical careers. Thus, the number of women applicants has increased by more than 300 percent since 1971.

RACE AND NATIONALITY

Because of affirmative-action programs, the admission rate for minority groups is higher than it is for white Americans even though minority students have lower grades.

Of all the groups, the Mexican Americans have the best chances of getting in. More than 51 percent of them were admitted as compared to only 37 percent of the white applicants. All of the other minority groups did better than the white American population. The acceptance rate was 41 percent for blacks and 43 percent for American Indians and mainland Puerto Ricans.

The average undergraduate grades for the minority applicants were far below the 3.28 GPA for white Americans. Black applicants had only a 2.70 GPA; American Indians, 2.98; Mexican-Americans, 2.91; and mainland Puerto Ricans, 3.13.

SOCIO-ECONOMIC BACKGROUND

The chances of getting into medical school steadily increase with the amount of money the applicant's parents make. Applicants from the highest "parental income" categories are almost 50 percent more likely to be accepted than those from the lowest categories.

The consistency of this correlation is shocking. With only one exception, each income category did better than the one preceding it in the 1975–76 study of applicants. The acceptance rate was:

33.8 percent for applicants in the "under $5,000" parental income
category
36.3 percent for $5,000 to $9,999
38.5 percent for $10,000 to $11,999
38.4 percent for $12,000 to $14,999 (This income category is the
only break in the correlation.)
41.5 percent for $15,000 to $19,999
43.5 percent for $20,000 to $24,999
46 percent for $25,000 to $49,999
47.9 percent for $50,000 or more a year

This is not, however, as sinister as it might at first appear. Undergraduate grades and college admission scores are also correlated with
parental income. At least in this study they were correlated up to the top
income group, where the correlation broke down.

Applicants whose families were in the $50,000 or more income cate-
gory did seem to have an advantage over other applicants. Their acceptance rate was the highest of all categories, though their grades and MCAT
scores were bested by applicants from less affluent families. But this may
be because there seems to be a prejudice in favor of the children of physicians, who also tend to be in the highest income categories.

The acceptance rate for the offspring of physicians was 43.2 percent as
compared to only 36.3 percent for the other occupation categories. They
achieved this higher rate even though their undergraduate grades were not
the best.

In fact the GPAs of the physicians' children were the eighth lowest of
ten categories studied. Having higher GPAs were children whose fathers
were in "other health occupations"; "other professions"; "ownership,
managerial, or administrative positions"; "clerical or sales work"; "craftsmanship, skilled work"; "farming"; or "other occupations."

A higher percentage of physicians' children, however, did take MCATs
and got better scores than the children in all the other categories except
"other professions."

UNDERGRADUATE MAJOR

It would appear that the best way to prepare for medical school is to major
in chemistry, biology, or other medically related fields as an undergraduate.
Though the majority of successful medical school applicants do just that,
majoring in these subjects does not give them much of an advantage over
the competition. Only 34.1 percent of the biology majors and 43.1 percent
of the chemistry majors were accepted as compared to an overall average
of 36.3 percent.

In fact, some of the nonmedical majors gave the applicants a slight advantage. The AAMC found that 52.8 percent of the applicants who majored in interdisciplinary fields were accepted, as were 49.2 percent of philosophy majors and 45.1 percent of anthropology majors.

The lowest acceptance rates were among students majoring in other professional fields. Only 19.1 percent of education majors and 26.4 percent of business majors were accepted. A surprisingly poor performance was turned in by students who majored in the paramedical fields. The acceptance rate for nursing was 23.3 percent; medical technology, 21.8 percent; and pharmacy, the lowest of all, 17.9 percent.

The AAMC concluded that on the average there was little correlation with undergraduate majors and success in getting into medical school.

□ □ □

James Nestor had worked harder than he ever had in his life to get good grades because he wanted to overcome the considerable odds against him and get into medical school. By the time he was through he had achieved an almost perfect 3.9 GPA in pre-med and MCAT scores in the 700s, which is about the best anyone can do. But even so things looked bad for Jim.

His advisers had told him that at thirty-five he was just too old to consider beginning a medical career. Only 18 percent of applicants between thirty-two and thirty-seven succeed. He was a mechanical engineer. Less than 30 percent of applicants with this major are accepted. And he had already been rejected by twenty-seven of the twenty-eight medical schools he had applied to.

Penn was the only school that hadn't rejected him yet. And this was the school he had wanted to get into most. Even living as far away as California, Jim was very much aware of Penn's liberal academic program. Jim did not want to take a regimented, by-the-numbers academic program. He was too old for that sort of nonsense. Penn was one of the few medical schools that had abandoned the more traditional and rigid approach to medical education.

And Penn had been the only school to offer Jim any kind of encouragement at all. The admissions committee had sent him a letter shortly after his interview saying that he was a good candidate and that they were holding his application for a second review at a later date.

That meant that Penn was putting his name on an alternate list should some of the students already accepted by the school decide not to come. It didn't seem likely that many would turn down the opportunity. And it seemed even more unlikely that anything would come of the Penn possibility now that four months had passed since the interview.

Jim was girding himself for the likelihood of soon returning to his engineering profession. After taking off for more than a year to study pre-med, it was going to be very disappointing to go back. To make the backward transition less painful, Jim decided to use up the few dollars he still had left and take a long vacation in Europe.

All summer long, Jim and his wife, Becky, traveled through the countryside of Europe. They felt the different cultures, moved with the different tempos of the cities and drank the wine. There was no tight itinerary. They just kept going, trying to stretch the money as far as possible. The geographical distance and the impact of the different cultures were making the United States and the medical school defeats seem far away.

They were in Luxembourg when the money ran out. It was no problem. They would take a plane back to the United States the next day. Since there was no telephone in their room, they went to the post office and Becky called some friends back home to tell them that they would soon be returning.

Jim was watching her as she spoke on the telephone, and the sudden look of shock on Becky's face scared him. *Someone has died,* he thought. He asked Becky what was wrong, but she shook her head.

"Here, you talk," she said, thrusting the telephone at him.

Anxiously, he took the phone and asked what was wrong. But the voice of the woman on the phone didn't sound scared. The connection was beautiful and the woman sounded happy and excited.

"Guess where you'll be living next fall," the voice yelled.

"What?" Jim asked, perplexed.

"I've been frantic, trying to get you all week," the voice said, ignoring the question. "You have only two weeks to answer the letter. Guess where you're going to be living next year."

"What are you talking about?" Jim asked again, confused now because Becky was looking at him with a huge smile and tears were welling in her eyes.

"You'll be living in Philadelphia," the voice shouted. "You've been accepted. The University of Pennsylvania has accepted you. You're going to go to medical school."

□ □ □

And so throughout the winter, spring, and summer of 1974 the letters of acceptance went out from Penn, and slowly the class of '78 was formed. Among the other students who would make up the class were:

Mark Reber, twenty-eight, a teacher of retarded children. A softspoken, sensitive man with a reddish beard and thick glasses, Mark would find the youthful competitiveness of his compulsive classmates harsh. But his gentleness would serve him well in dealing with sick children and he would become convinced that he had made the right choice in picking pediatrics as a specialty.

Steven Levine, married, thirty years old, and a Ph.D. in clinical psychology. Steve had already started a practice in Los Angeles, but closed it down in preference for a career in medicine. An unusually emotionally aware person, Steve would find the physical aspects of death difficult to deal with at first.

Helene Silverblatt, twenty-six, a bilingual anthropologist who once taught English to Puerto Ricans in north Philadelphia. She decided to become a physician because she was appalled by the inadequate medical treatment Puerto Ricans were getting. A Marxist in political philosophy and very socially conscious, she would have trouble identifying with the middle-class mentality of her classmates and frequently would long to be with the Peruvian peasants she had come to know as an anthropologist.

Walter Tsou, twenty-one, chemistry major at Penn and the son of a chemistry professor there. Since high school, Walter had wanted to become a physician, and he worked diligently toward that goal. He laughed easily, wore University of Pennsylvania Streaking Team shirts, and joked often. But underneath he was anxious about the prospects of medical school. When he talked about such things, his legs and hands were in constant, nervous motion.

Barbara Turner, twenty-four, master's degree in fine arts from Harvard University. She chose medicine because she wanted a "vitally alive" field where she would have human contact and a strong feeling of accomplishment.

Daniel O. Dadda, thirty, married to a Nigerian princess, father of one child. His father was a retired headmaster of a school in Nigeria. Daniel also was a headmaster. He would spend at least seven years in the United States learning how to be a physician and then return home to a country where almost all of the people went to the voodoo doctor because there weren't enough western-trained physicians.

Ronald Cargill, twenty-four, engaged, biology major. His father was a civilian naval equipment specialist. Ronald was a member of the Black Muslims, a black religious and social sect that preached separatism from whites. Part of Ronald's education was being paid for by the Black Muslims and he would spend weekends during medical school preaching the faith on ghetto street corners.

Of the 160 students who would gather together for the first time in September, two would withdraw during the first year for medical reasons and a third would leave a year later because she didn't like medicine.

All the others, however, would successfully go through the demanding, frequently exhausting, sometimes scary business of becoming a physician. They would work seventy-, eighty- and ninety-hour weeks. They would deliver babies, witness death, and learn to use the pain of patients as a diagnostic tool rather than shrink from it.

In the coming years, they would cut into human skin with scalpels and then sew it back together again with needle and thread. They would assist at operations, help to revive the dying in emergency situations, and learn to deal with the grief of relatives who could not understand how man, God, or nature could be so cruel.

They would experience the pride, but more often the discomfort, of being imbued with Godlike qualities by naïve patients. They would also feel the anger of people when medical science failed. They would be impressed by the incredible things medicine could do. But they would also be depressed and frightened by the extent of its limitations.

All of the students, at one time or another, would experience the intense loneliness of a student who tries to master mountains of material. They would feel inadequate and unsure. And many times they would question the decision to become a physician.

But when it was all over, this tortuous educational process would have turned them from laymen into physicians. Few would realize how much all of this would change them as people, but to the rest of the world they would no longer be the same. They would be treated as people who were a little special.

And wherever they went, people would address them as "Doctor."

2

The morning was unusually humid for September and the antiquated amphitheater in the University of Pennsylvania School of Medicine was not air-conditioned.

The damp discomfort made their clothes stick to the backs of the medical students who began to fill the graduated tiers of seats. The first-year students tried to look casual as though this were just another morning in another lecture hall, only one more step in a lengthy educational process that already had taken seventeen or eighteen years.

Rikki Lights had taken a seat way in the back of the large room and spoke to no one. After having attended a women's college for four years, it felt strange to sit in a room predominantly filled with males. She was glad to see the few black students that she did.

Jim Nestor sat a few rows down from Rikki's high perch. Even though everyone seemed nervously talkative, Jim sensed a sincere effort to make contact. But he was also very much aware of how young everyone else was, and thirty-five felt very old to him.

Matt Lotysh sat talking to his new roommate, another medical student, who would share the rent on a small townhouse across the river from the medical school. And Randy Wiest surveyed the room filling with people, wondering if any of them liked the outdoors. He didn't know it, but there was one student who did like camping as much as he did. He would marry her within the year.

As the hour approached, more and more students came rushing through the doors of the amphitheater, out of breath or confused from having gotten lost. There was the hushed mumbling of some people talking, but most of the students, still strangers to one another, sat quietly staring down he rows of seats.

Finally, a few minutes after nine, a short man with glasses and a conservative dark business suit walked down the aisle to the speaker's pit, hooked the microphone around his neck, and looked up at the students sitting above him. It was Dr. Edward J. Stemmler, acting dean of the school of medicine.

Talk stopped abruptly. Dr. Stemmler smiled.

"I want to welcome you to medical school. It's obvious that you've come a long way . . . seven or eight years of a very competitive life has brought you here . . . but the competition is over now."

Some of the students smiled; others looked skeptical.

Dean Stemmler warned them that the coming years would be difficult ones and that at one time or another all of them would wonder if they had made the right choice in deciding to become physicians. He spoke about how lonely it would feel spending long nights trying to master huge amounts of complex material and wondering if they were equal to the task.

Six days a week would be spent in the laboratories and lecture halls for a total of thirty-eight hours, as compared to the sixteen hours of classwork an undergraduate takes. And on top of that would come the three or four hours of book work each night, making for sixty- to seventy-hour weeks.

But instead of trying to frighten them, Dean Stemmler reassured the students that they would do well because they had been carefully chosen. He told them not to worry about understanding everything, because there was just too much information to take in at once. Much of the medical education process is repetitive, he reassured the students. They would be exposed to the same information again and again in the coming four years and after a while all of the important information would be absorbed.

The reassuring theme that Dean Stemmler established was repeated by the other faculty members and upper classmen who followed him to the speaker's pit.

A handsome second-year student told the students to have fun in the coming years.

"Get out and make friends and lead a full life," he said, sounding more like a recruiter for a fraternity house than a medical student welcoming a new class.

"Don't study every hour of every night of the week," he said. "You're all going to do that at first. I know you will because that's what I did when I came here. But it will be a mistake. They're going to be throwing so much information at you that you'll be walking around in a daze if you don't set some limits. So don't try to do the impossible. Get out and date and do some jogging and have some fun. This is going to be a great time in your life."

Now the students were looking at one another with suspicion. These were strange things to hear on the first day of medical school when common sense would say that the competition was just beginning and that all pleasures should be put aside for the time being to permit hard work.

The more ambitious students, hardened by the ruthless competition of pre-med, didn't trust all these smiling people who had addressed them. They knew that in four years, when they graduated, only the top students would get into the best internship and residency programs. As far as they were concerned, the race was only half over despite what the dean had said. And in some ways they were right.

All the reassurance would have only a limited effect, and everyone who spoke the first day knew it. There was no question that the students would complete the work successfully—the selection process guaranteed that by admitting only the brightest and most strongly motivated. But, ironically, these very qualities also condemned these students to a frustration and loneliness that no amount of reassurance would relieve.

Accustomed to mastering all the material presented to them in undergraduate school and pre-med, they would try to do the same thing in medical school. But they wouldn't succeed this time, and it would take months of lonely frustration to realize that they shouldn't try.

After the orientation session, the students had box lunches with the upper classmen on the lawns outside. The warm sun felt good, even in the humid air. It was Tuesday. Classes would not start for real until Thursday.

The students spent Wednesday walking around the campus, getting keys to microscope lockers and buying books and white coats at Dolbey's, the medical bookstore on campus. Downtown Philadelphia, just across the river, couldn't have looked lovelier than it did this fall month. It was the calm before the storm of study.

The excitement of discovering a new city and new people was overwhelmed by the realization that they were finally entering the medical profession. They were crossing the line that separated laymen from the physician. Now they would learn about medicine from the other end of the stethoscope.

They had won the right to understand the mystery behind the medical rituals. They would find out all the things the little black bag contained and how to use the potions and charms. They would learn the meaning of the shadows on the x-ray films and discover all the secret things that happen in the operating rooms and laboratories and morgue.

Being among the privileged, they would be permitted in the small huddles of doctors and nurses at the foot of the hospital bed, out of earshot of patients, relatives, and others not in the fraternity. They would bring life into the world. And they would see it leave.

No phase of the initiation rites would be more jarring to the novitiates than confronting death for the first time—not as distant observers with sideway glances, but as participants in the process. Rather than being shielded from death by social taboos, medical students must see and smell it, touch it, cut into it. The first day in anatomy class, when students are required to confront the yellow, waxy form of a dead human body, is a scary and memorable experience.

For the class of '78 there was no preparation for this moment because it came on Thursday, the first full day of school, early in the morning before lunch. The students were shocked by the suddenness of their plunge into the business of becoming physicians.

□ □ □

The anatomy laboratory was at the end of a hall in one of the oldest medical school buildings. It was a brightly lit room with low-hanging fluorescent lights and frosted windows to keep the curious from peering in. And everywhere was the smell of the chemicals used to preserve the bodies.

Usually a class enters a room en masse with a lot of talking and laughing. But the first time the students entered the autopsy lab they did so quietly with the reverence usually inspired by death.

Twenty-eight bodies, shrouded in tightly wrapped plastic covers that revealed the shapes of the enclosed cadavers, lay on stone-covered dissecting tables. Heavily embalmed to prevent deterioration, the bodies would remain on these tables until final exams at Christmas time.

The age, sex, and cause of death of each body was listed by table number on the bulletin board next to the door of the lab. There were nineteen males and nine females. They all had died in 1973 and ranged in age from forty-five to ninety-three.

Six students were assigned to each table. They stood quietly with their new dissecting kits, purchased at Dolbey's, waiting for the instructor to tell them what to do. There were only five students at Steve's table because Steve hadn't arrived yet.

One of the five, a younger student, looked at the mound and shook his head. "Boy, I hope our body isn't fat," he said with an attempt to sound knowledgeable about such things. "My brother is a fourth-year student and he said it's hell when they're fat because you're up to your elbows in grease."

The young student was greeted with contemptuous glances by his teammates who then regarded the large form before them. The names of all the people at Steve's table began with the letter L because assignments to the tables were done alphabetically. Friends in medical school frequently have the same last initial because many friendships begin at the dissecting table where students spend three mornings a week working very close together, exploring their first body together as a team.

Six students are a lot for one cadaver, but bodies for anatomy class have become scarce. Only a few years ago, most of the cadavers were the unclaimed bodies of the poor who died unwanted in the charity wards of hospitals. But conditions have improved, and today there are not enough unclaimed bodies, so 50 percent of the cadavers are willed. At the end of the semester the remains are cremated and buried in a mass burial site after multidenominational funeral services are conducted.

"Okay, you can start unwrapping the bodies now." It was the instructor, an older man in a long white lab coat, standing at the end of the room. There was little talk and only the bustle of students unwrapping the plastic shrouds could be heard. Steve arrived in the middle of this, fifteen minutes late. He found his table and took his place with his team, which had just exposed the body of an eighty-one-year-old woman who presumably had died of natural causes. She was very fat. Some of the students sighed, looking at their young colleague who had warned them about such things.

Briefly the anatomy professor explained how and where to make the first incision, warning them to be careful and to note each layer of tissue as they went through it. The purpose of the course was to lay bare the human body, painstakingly exposing and recognizing every muscle, nerve, organ, and bone. It would be a tedious process, requiring patience and a prodigious memory to remember the names, functions, and location of all the parts.

The professor finished his explanation and told the class to begin. Taking the new scalpel from its case, Steve pressed the blade into the clear field of the yellowed skin of the woman's chest and pulled it along the incision line the team had agreed on. The blade was sharp and the skin parted easily, revealing a deep canyon of fat that looked surprisingly similar to the fat on a steak. The students had kept the plastic cover over the woman's face.

Each student took turns cutting into the cadaver while their teammates consulted the anatomy text with its sketches and descriptions of the landmarks in the human body. They worked quietly and intensely this first morning. It would become noisier as the semester progressed and the students became more casual about the dead.

Walter Tsou was dissecting the frail thin body of a fifty-five-year-old pneumonia victim. Helene Silverblatt's cadaver was an eighty-one-year-old black man. It wasn't until midway through the morning that she noticed the bulletin board and discovered that her cadaver had died of exposure. It was ironic that of all the bodies this one should be assigned to Helene, a woman who had entered medicine partly because she was appalled by the deplorable health conditions of the poor.

From that moment, the body on the table was no longer a cadaver to Helene, but an old man who had died of neglect. It was several days before the thought would go.

The class spent the morning cutting through the skin and fat and fascia in and around the muscles of their cadavers. It was slow going because it was hard to differentiate the anatomical structures, which appeared so clearly in the sketches of the anatomy textbook but were lost amid the clutter of tissue that constituted the real human body. Finally the morning was over. Happily rewrapping the bodies, the students packed away their scalpels, locked their now stained and smelly white lab coats in their steel lockers, and left this room for lunch, where they talked about all that they had just experienced.

Steve didn't feel like lunch, but instead went off to the cafeteria of the University of Pennsylvania Hospital for coffee.

"All our lives we're taught to respect the human body," he said, fingering the cup of coffee. "I never stabbed anyone in my life, but today I picked up a scalpel and pushed it through human skin."

He was glad that this confrontation he had been dreading for so long was over now, but in some ways the bad thoughts were clinging more than he would have liked. And now there was the other fear to deal with, one that bothers medical students even more than their first cadaver: observing an autopsy. Here the body would be more life-like than the one- or two-year-old cadavers.

It would be another week before the class attended an autopsy, and Steve was anxious to get this over with also.

□ □ □

Many of the students in the class of '78 formed their attitudes toward society and the medical establishment during the late sixties and early seventies. These were the years of protest marches, antiwar demonstrations, and consciousness-raising folk songs.

Inspired by such things, the new, socially aware student came to Penn determined not to be perverted by medical school or the medical establishment. He would not become indifferent to the social needs of his patients. He would speak out against any hint of racism, elitism, chauvinism, or any of the other isms that subordinated one human being to another.

In the first few days of medical school these students did see some callousness on the part of the faculty and their fellow students. Sometimes what they saw as callousness was merely the result of their own excessive sensitivity. Other times they were right.

In introducing a class to the cadaver for the first time, one of the instructors casually rested his hand on the deceased's chest, to the annoyance of some students.

A few days later a surgeon advised the students to pay particular attention to the dissection of a particular nerve. Offhandedly he remarked that as a student he had not done his homework and subsequently in practice severed the nerve by mistake, making it forever impossible for the patient to lift his hand very high.

What nettled some watchers was not that he had made a mistake, but the matter-of-fact way in which the doctor told how his mistake had crippled another human for life.

All week long doctors were trooping into pathology class from one hospital or another with a display of what they termed "fresh pathology," which consisted of assortments of organs from people who had died a few hours earlier.

The more sensitive students turned to their peers for support, but often they met indifference or contempt for being so silly as to be concerned about extraneous considerations.

The adjustment to these realities was difficult, and the students got lit-

tle help in sorting out their feelings. Penn had tried to make the educational process less traumatic with a new curriculum, started six years
earlier. Emphasis was placed on making the educational experience more
humane and flexible to counteract the pressure-cooker conditioning of
undergraduate school and pre-med, where two points in a cumulative
average could determine whether or not a student became a doctor, and
all peers were enemies trying to cheat him out of his career.

Under the new curriculum, every Thursday afternoon the students
would be given a clinical introductory course designed to make them
aware of patients and their needs as people. On these days the students
would put on their white coats and go to the hospitals where they'd meet
patients and get medical histories. The purpose of this was to make the
students aware of the fact that all the abstract knowledge they were acquiring eventually would be applied to human beings. In the old days students
wouldn't get a chance to see a real-live patient until the third year.

Penn also tried to make courses, class requirements, and procedures
less rigid and competitive in keeping with the more liberal climate.

In pathology class, for instance, professors would take attendance, but
they would do it only to get to know the students and no records would be
kept. Students were advised to cut class if they were bored or had something more useful to do.

Some textbooks were recommended, but students could read whatever
they wanted to cover the subject material. Final exams were required, but
the grades were only pass, fail, or honors. Quizzes would be given during
the semester, but only if the students requested them to identify their weak
areas, and again no records would be kept.

And all the time students would be reminded that they could not
learn everything, so relax.

The seemingly casual, uncompetitive atmosphere the medical school
tried to impose sounded like an undergraduate's dream come true. But it
was disconcerting to these compulsive students. They were suspicious of it.
And they weren't going to be fooled.

□ □ □

Randy spent Friday evening studying in his Graduate Towers apartment
overlooking the Penn campus. The upper classmen had said that three
hours of study a night was enough, but already Randy could see that three
hours wouldn't do. Five hours a night, at least, he thought, plus a few
hours over the weekend. This annoyed him because it did not leave any
time for jogging or camping, but he felt that he had better apply himself to
his studies.

While Randy was poring over his books in Graduate Towers, Helene
was having dinner with a new friend at La Terrasse, a French restaurant
on the Penn campus. The talk was about medical school and anthropology,

but mostly Helene spoke of Sarhua and the people there she had come to love.

The village could be reached only by an eight-hour walk along the trails. The fifteen hundred people of Sarhua were all farmers who worked hard in the daytime and who, at the slightest provocation—like a wedding or the closing of a business deal—would spend the evening singing, dancing, and drinking.

The people were very open and loving, she said, and the dramatic Andes were beautiful, but disease was rampant and the prenatal death rate was terribly high. One of Helene's hopes was to return as a doctor for several months and provide some basic medical training for the people.

The wine with dinner and the talk of Sarhua made Helene feel warm. She had not started studying yet, but there would be enough time for that later. Medical school was starting well for her. She was filled with good memories from the summer. And the sky was bright with stars as she walked through the small park near her commune on Forty-fifth Street.

"*Bonita Andahuaylas, porque te quiero tanto, te adoro tanto,*" she sang in Spanish, filling the night with a lilting romantic melody. ("Pretty woman from Andahuaylas, why do I love you so much, adore you so much? Because in this world of Humanga, there is so much beauty.")

Sunday was one of those beautiful crisp fall days that made living in the Northeast worth it all. The air was clear and the coldness was just enough to suggest fall. The city was awakening from the summer doldrums.

□ □ □

Steve slept late that morning, having stayed awake the night before talking to house guests he and his wife, Laura, were entertaining over the weekend. It was just as well because he hadn't been sleeping well ever since school started.

Barbara Turner had been up for hours. She was visiting a friend of her mother's in Swarthmore and started Sunday morning by reading a chapter on the cardiovascular system.

Meanwhile, in Philadelphia, an old black man lay in a bed in the Veterans' Administration hospital, fighting the cancer that had taken over his body. He would be dead before Barbara finished the chapter and before Steve woke up.

They would all come together the next morning when Barbara and Steve's section of the pathology class were sent to the VA hospital to witness the first autopsy anyone in the class had seen.

Autopsies are an invaluable part of medicine and medical education. By performing autopsies, physicians can determine the accuracy of their diagnoses and the effectiveness of their treatment, hopefully to the advantage of patients to follow.

First-year medical students are required to attend at least one autopsy.

Supposedly it helps them better understand the workings of the human body, the relationship of organs, and the disease process. More likely its only true impact is to impress them with the reality of death.

□ □ □

The pathology lecture started Monday with the announcement that the first section would be attending an autopsy that morning at the VA hospital.

After the lecture was over, Steve and Barbara walked together to the hospital. Neither was looking forward to this moment, and they found comfort in each other's company.

The average physician will see much death and countless bodies, which he will forget in the course of his career. But every doctor remembers that first autopsy just as he remembers his first day in anatomy class and the first time he delivers a baby.

The body of the old man lay naked on a stainless-steel autopsy table, his head propped up by a wooden block.

Morgue assistant Rubin Whitehead planned to do a Rokytanski procedure on the body. This is a widely performed method in which the viscera are detached from the shell of the body in such a way that all the organs from the small intestines to the windpipe can be removed as a single unit, attached to one another. This enables the pathologist to dissect the organs on a table away from the body.

The ten students clustered around the table as Whitehead worked efficiently, joking as he went along. He thought that this relieved the tension, but it didn't.

Walter Tsou, who dealt with tension by laughing, was laughing almost constantly now. Steve was markedly pale. And Barbara stood to the rear of the group of students. Many of the others cupped the fronts of their surgical gowns over their noses because of the odor.

The small group that had crowded closer and closer around the table as Whitehead worked jerked back in alarm and gasped. Whitehead had reached into the body and pulled out all of the organs in a single connected mass, like bananas on a stalk.

The viscera were turned over to the pathologist who cut through the fat and other tissue, exposing the individual organs in search of disease. Doctors never know the full extent of the disease in the patients they are treating because they can make only inferences on the basis of lab tests, x-rays, and symptoms.

The old man's lungs were black from a lifetime of breathing city air. The bronchus leading to the lungs was cut open with scissors and again the students gasped. The pathologist had revealed white nodules that looked like bright pebbles clogging a pipe.

All their lives these students had heard of lung cancer, but never had they seen it. Now there it was before them on the autopsy table.

With a large blade that looked more like a butcher knife than a surgical instrument, the pathologist cut into the blackened lungs. More white nodules were exposed. He cut into another lobe and found still more. The man's lungs were filled with cancer.

All the students had moved over to the small dissecting sink, crowding around the pathologist, who was working under the bright light from the overhead surgical lamp. No longer of interest, the body lay on a stainless-steel table by itself, a towel draped over the face, as though all the activity at the nearby sink had nothing to do with it.

To the medically naïve students it seemed ironic that the human form should have so little interest to the pathologist. He cared little about the eyes and nose and lips, which in life expressed the most human quality— the personality of the individual.

Instead the pathologist was interested in the heart and liver and lungs and kidneys and the other hidden structures that supported life. It was here that he would find the disease that had progressed silently and unnoticed for so many years until it took the life of its host.

With a scalpel the pathologist cut into the old man's coronary arteries and exposed a firm white fibrous material that had severely narrowed the opening of the vessels. It was severe atherosclerosis. If the cancer hadn't killed him, the old man would have probably soon been struck down by a heart attack.

The old man's heart was held in the pathologist's gloved hand. Surrounded by fat and other tissue, it didn't look at all familiar. It didn't even remotely resemble the organ depicted on Valentine cards. Cutting into the heart, the pathologist showed the pumping chambers to the students crowded around him.

The lifeless tissue seemed no more impressive than meat on a butcher's block. Yet only hours earlier this heart had been beating as steadily as it had for seventy-five years, keeping an old man alive until the cancer killed him.

Of all the organs scattered about on the dissecting table, the only ones that were easily recognizable were the shiny brownish red kidneys, and then only because they resembled the beans that were named after them.

As the autopsy progressed, some of the students became braver and more accustomed to the smells of chemicals and cancerous tissue. They stopped shielding their noses with their coats and moved closer to the table. The pathologist asked for assistance in holding the kidney he was about to dissect. He didn't really need help but wanted to challenge the students' courage. A woman student immediately offered and put on a surgeon's gloves, taking care not to grimace or smile.

Confronting fresh death was disturbing to those students who could not rid themselves of the conventional, romanticized view of human life. To accept an autopsy without emotional trauma, it is necessary to see the organs and bodies and faces as merely lifeless tissue with no more claim to revered human status than any other biologic material.

But such romanticism is not easily shed, and many of the students couldn't help but think of their own hearts and livers and lungs when they saw the old man's organs on the table, pitifully bare and vulnerable. It was so shocking to think that human organs were not special, that they looked like the meat in a butcher shop and in some ways were treated like that by the pathologist.

The students had been in the morgue only an hour, but it seemed much longer because they had been so alert to everything that was happening. It was not a particularly interesting case for the pathologist because the disease process was obvious and didn't require particular skill on the part of the specialist. Finishing what he was doing, the pathologist confirmed what the old man's physician had known anyhow. Cause of death was lung cancer. The students managed a smile, thanked the pathologist, and left.

Steve spent his lunchtime sitting on the stone wall outside the medical school building under the trees along Hamilton Walk. A half-eaten sandwich lay next to him. For many minutes he just stared ahead, saying nothing to the people around him.

"Boy, this transition sure is hard."

Steve looked up. It was Barbara, who had just come from the bookstore with Walter.

Barbara was still stunned from the sharp transition. At one moment she was standing in the morgue in front of a body being dissected. Then minutes later she was standing in a bookstore with laughing students who never had seen such a thing and were unaware of what just had happened in the morgue a few hundred yards away.

"Do you realize what we have seen in only two weeks?" Walter said, still emotionally high from the experience. "I find the whole thing so exciting, I can't believe that it's all happening."

Steve studied Walter hard for several moments.

An art student hurried down the walk, a blank canvas under his arm. A group of laughing and joking undergraduates ambled by. And the thumping beat of a rock record came through the open window of a dormitory opposite the medical school.

The beautiful weather that had arrived over the weekend was still around, and the bright sunlight in the clear air lit up the leaves in a thousand different shades of green.

3

Wearing new short white coats that made them feel self-conscious, the twenty students crowded outside the office of the chief medical resident, waiting for him to arrive.

They had been in medical school only three weeks, yet in a few minutes they would meet their first hospital patient. They wouldn't touch the patient or even talk to him much, but symbolically the encounter would be important.

It would mark the first time the students stood on the other side of the line in the doctor-patient relationship. When they had been inside hospitals before it had always been as patients or visitors—outsiders who could only wonder what went on behind the scenes. Now they would begin to find out.

The students were unusually talkative this particular day. It was obvious that they were nervous, not because they were about to meet the patient but because they were wearing the white coat for the first time.

As symbols of office go, the short white coat is not particularly impressive. It is made of cheap cotton with extra large pockets to accommodate the books, examining kits, stethoscopes, and other paraphernalia that students carry with them. They wrinkle easily. And the tailoring is notoriously poor.

But to everyone who works in a teaching hospital—from the janitor and orderlies to the highest-ranking research physician—the short white coat signifies one thing—MEDICAL STUDENT! The students wouldn't be more conspicuous if they wore signs and beat drums.

It was well after 2:00 P.M. now, the time they were supposed to meet the resident, but he still hadn't showed up. This in itself was a lesson for the students, who would repeatedly discover that they didn't rank high on the list of priorities in busy city hospitals. If duties conflicted and something had to give, invariably the busy house staff physician would reschedule the meeting with the students or arrive late or simply not show up.

Helene arrived a few minutes late. She smiled to a couple of students with whom she had become friendly and took her folded white coat out of her red canvas book bag.

Many of the students enjoyed walking down Hamilton Walk past the undergraduate dormitories to the VA hospital wearing the coat. For them this had status.

But in Helene's circle of friends, political ideals and social causes were the important things, not symbols of authority or social prestige, so she preferred not to wear her coat until inside the hospital, where it was required. Putting the coat on, she pulled her long black hair from under the collar and allowed it to fall down her back.

While the students waited, the patient they were about to meet, fifty-five-year-old Joseph Insolia, played solitaire in a sixteen-bed ward a few hundred feet down the hall.

Mr. Insolia, a Collingdale electrician, had been admitted to the Veterans' Administration hospital two weeks previously with a suspected heart attack. His condition improved after a stay in the hospital, and now the doctors were checking him for a few other things before releasing him.

During rounds that morning, the chief resident told Mr. Insolia about the student doctors coming in that afternoon and asked him if he minded going before them as a sample patient. Mr. Insolia agreed readily. Actually the idea delighted the easy-going electrician, who was getting bored sitting around the hospital.

He liked talking about his symptoms. And that a roomful of student doctors would be discussing his illness made his medical problem seem unique, if not historic. Mr. Insolia would go back home and tell his friends that he had had such an unusual medical problem that twenty new doctors were called in just to consider it.

Actually the University of Pennsylvania School of Medicine had little interest in Mr. Insolia's heart trouble as such. The purpose of the impending encounter was to demonstrate to the students the proper method of getting a medical history from a patient.

Mr. Insolia would sit before the class and answer questions as the chief resident went through the process of getting the history, explaining to the students each step as he did it. The resident would pretend that he didn't already know what was wrong with Mr. Insolia, and the students, who wouldn't know the diagnosis either, would experience the excitement of solving a diagnostic mystery.

□ □ □

The chief medical resident, Dr. Stanley Goldfarb, arrived at 2:30, precisely a half hour late. Trailing a long, flowing white coat that was the symbol of his higher rank in the hospital, Dr. Goldfarb hurried down the hall to the waiting students, announced that he would give them a briefing in a room nearby, and turned again, the contingent of suddenly quieted students in pursuit.

The first room Dr. Goldfarb looked into was filled with nurses holding a meeting, so he reversed himself and found an empty room at the other end of the hall. Sitting down on a folding chair at the front of the room, Dr. Goldfarb got ready to speak as the students filed into the room and took their places in classroom chairs equipped with armboards for taking notes.

"Hello, I'm Dr. Stanley Goldfarb, the chief medical resident here at the VA," Dr. Goldfarb said. "I wanted to talk to you for a few minutes before we bring the patient in so you'll understand what we'll be doing.

"At the outset I want to remind you that as student doctors you will be getting privileged information from the patients you come in contact with and that you should respect this."

A few of the students sneaked glances at one another and smiled. They were crossing the line that separated the rest of the world from the private inner sanctum of the medical profession.

A late-arriving student stuck his head in the door, recognized his classmates, and quickly found a seat. Dr. Goldfarb watched him and then resumed his lecture.

"The purpose of the medical history is, of course, to find out what is wrong with the patient, but you can't do this by bombarding him with a barrage of questions," Dr. Goldfarb said. "First you have to establish a relationship with him and he must have the opportunity to establish one with you. If he doesn't like you or distrusts you because you are indifferent to him as a person, you're not going to get anywhere no matter how much you know about medicine.

"Start off the interview by introducing yourself and asking how the patient feels," Dr. Goldfarb continued. "This isn't a social amenity. It's a very important part of the process because it gives you a chance to establish personal contact with the patient and it shows him that you are concerned about him as a person.

"You start collecting important information the moment you see the patient—even before he has said a word. What is his skin color? Is he breathing rapidly? Shaking hands may reveal all sorts of things. Is his hand cold and moist, indicating anxiety? Is it the weak grasp of a feeble person or the powerful handshake of someone trying to deny illness? Does he have the bewildered expression of someone who is demented?"

Dr. Goldfarb continued along these lines for several minutes as the students became increasingly anxious to see this information put into practice with the patient.

□ □ □

With all the publicity given to esoteric electronic equipment, daring surgery, and miracle drugs, few people realize that the single most important thing a doctor does in diagnosing illness and providing care is getting a detailed medical history.

Few diseases are so straightforward that they can be definitively diagnosed with a single laboratory study or x-ray, and even in those cases where this is possible, a medical history is needed first to know which tests to order.

In obtaining a medical history, the skillful physician will ask questions in such an unimposing manner that the patient doesn't realize how complex a process it is. He has no idea how much training went into learning how to conduct the interview so that clues to illness aren't missed because the patient mistakenly believes that an important symptom isn't worth mentioning.

No two physicians obtain a medical history in exactly the same way because they adapt the technique to their personalities and the manner in which they relate to their patients. But most physicians will follow certain basic principles.

Since the patient is primarily concerned about the problem that brought him to the physician or the hospital in the first place, the doctor begins his history-taking session by focusing on the present illness.

At first the questions are kept purposely broad so that the patient has a chance to express himself freely. A long list of precise questions tends to discourage the patient from volunteering information that might be important.

The medically naïve patient thinks a doctor can diagnose illness on the basis of a single symptom, but the mere statement that "my belly hurts" or "I keep getting this pain in my chest" means little by itself.

The physician looks for a constellation of symptoms—a syndrome—that might suggest a particular disease. Rarely does a malfunctioning organ or a disease produce only a single symptom. Pneumonia, for instance, doesn't result only in coughing or chest pain, it also causes a fever, sweating, and a loss of appetite.

Abdominal pain could mean a thousand things. If the pain is sharply localized underneath or just below the breast bone so that the patient can point to the exact spot where it hurts, that could mean an active ulcer.

Alternatively, if the abdominal pain comes on suddenly in the lower half of the belly and is accompanied by vomiting and diarrhea, food poisoning would be more likely. An inflamed gall bladder frequently has a slow buildup of pain, while kidney stones will produce sudden sharp pain in the flanks radiating to the lower abdomen.

But rarely does the patient describe the symptoms in such detail that the physician doesn't have to pursue the symptomatic clues with a line of questions like a detective interviewing witnesses at the scene of a crime.

Pain is the most frequent symptom, and the physician will ask a series of questions to determine where the pain is located, how intense it is, what the patient does to make it worse or better, how the pain developed over a period of hours or weeks, and so on.

Answers to these questions help determine the cause. But it's not as straightforward as it might appear. For instance, the thing that is broken or malfunctioning is not necessarily the thing that hurts. Pain may precisely indicate where someone might have cut themselves or been burned, but pain from internal organs is more complex to interpret. Unlike the skin, which is a blanket of nerves, the inner structures of the body are not so well supplied with nerves, and the pain might travel down neurologic pathways, popping up in strange places.

Pain radiating down the left arm to the elbow might have nothing to do with the limb itself, but mean that the patient is suffering a heart attack. On the other hand if the limb pain is associated with moving the affected arm, chances are good that it's caused by a muscle problem. Throbbing pain—such as from a migraine headache—is caused by the arteries painfully responding to the blood being pulsed through the body.

Some pain is almost, but not completely, revealing. For instance, severe pain in the big toe strongly suggests gout, though physical injury could do the same thing, and, conversely, gout can affect other joints.

Sometimes the association of pain is obvious. If the gastrointestinal tract is damaged or diseased, the pain frequently increases with eating and lessens with fasting. If the pain is relieved by drawing up the legs to the chest while lying in bed, this might suggest that something is wrong with the pancreas, because such a maneuver relieves the pressure on this organ, though the fetal position is comforting for all manner of problems.

Once the physician is confident that he has obtained all the information he can on the symptoms and the extent of the present illness, he moves on to the four other major categories of the interview:

Past health, involving a general appraisal of the patient's health prior to the present illness.

Family health, covering the immediate family and close relatives.

Social history, including such things as marital relations and job stress.

Systems review, which checks out each of the major organ systems of the body.

To the patient, all of this might appear irrelevant, especially if he came to see the doctor for a particular problem rather than for a general checkup. But each of these phases of the interview contributes to an understanding of the patient, if not the present illness.

For instance, a patient who is being treated for a heart attack might tell the doctor that his past health has been excellent except that he strained his chest muscles six months earlier, causing pain that spread to his arm. Since these are the classic symptoms of a heart attack, such a report would suggest that the patient had unknowingly suffered a previous heart attack and that the heart disease had been progressing for a while.

The family history might reveal that brothers, sisters, or parents had died of heart trouble, indicating a genetic component in the patient's current medical problem.

And the social history could show stresses at home or on the job that were aggravating the heart condition.

The review of systems is a backstop for the physician, who might miss unrelated but important symptoms during the first part of the interview when generalities were being discussed.

Usually starting with the skin and head, and working downward, the physician will ask the patient such questions as:

"Are you bothered by facial pain or headaches?"

"Do you have deafness or pain in the ears?"

"Do you have sinus pain?"

"How are your teeth?"

"Have you felt any pain or lumps in the breasts?"

"Do you ever get chest pain?"

"Do you get out of breath easily?"

"Do you have a good appetite? Any abdominal pain?"

"Do you have nausea or do you vomit?"

"Any pain on urination?"

"Are you troubled by pain in your legs or other joints?"

The nervous system will be evaluated with questions about dizziness, speech difficulties, and vertigo.

And finally the review of systems will be brought to a close with a brief assessment of the patient's psychological status when the doctor asks questions about such things as nervousness, memory loss, and insomnia.

The review of systems may open up an entirely new line of inquiry for the doctor. Discovering that the patient does have headaches or pain upon urination or that he has lost his appetite and vomits frequently suggests many different things. The physician must rule out the possible causes one by one until he is left with only the most likely. This is called a differential diagnosis because one disease must be differentiated from another in making a diagnosis.

The physician considers a myriad of possibilities when he starts his differential with the initial symptom. Headaches are caused by such things as tension, brain tumors, meningitis, fevers, eye problems, head injuries, blood infections, sinus disease, sunstroke, and so on.

Even a syndrome is not necessarily specific for one disease. One of the most common syndromes—loss of appetite, vomiting, and nausea—may be caused by psychological or physical problems. A frequent cause is depression or fear. But then again obstruction of the GI tract will cause the same symptoms. So will drug poisoning, acute appendicitis, diabetes, Addison's disease, heart trouble, and malnutrition.

It was becoming clear to the students as Dr. Goldfarb went deeper into such considerations why good diagnosticians were considered artists.

□ □ □

Dr. Goldfarb finished his short lecture and asked the students if they had any questions. There weren't any, so Dr. Goldfarb went out and brought in Mr. Insolia, who had been waiting in a nearby room.

He was an obese man with a chubby smiling face and a balding head. He wore the flimsy light-blue bathrobe of the VA hospital. He didn't seem bothered by the students, who all turned to look at him as he came in, but instead walked with slow assurance to the front of the room, where he sat down in the chair offered to him by Dr. Goldfarb.

Dr. Goldfarb introduced him to the students and made some small talk to establish a relationship the way he had told the students to do. Finally he got down to the business of getting the medical history.

"What brought you to the hospital?" Dr. Goldfarb asked, and Mr. Insolia began the long story about how he had become sick, led along by the preordained line of questions.

Mr. Insolia was a good history-giver and answered the questions succinctly but fully, without digressions into medically unimportant trivia that annoy the rushed physician. Dr. Goldfarb gave Mr. Insolia freedom to express himself the way he wanted. He didn't zero in on anything until Mr. Insolia mentioned the pounding in his chest.

"When did you first notice this?" Dr. Goldfarb said abruptly.

"It was after work and I was walking to catch my train. I wasn't running or anything, just ambling along, looking forward to baseball on TV that night, when suddenly it hit me. Wham! Just like that."

"What hit you?" Dr. Goldfarb asked gently, with obvious concern.

"This terrible pounding in my chest. Bam! Bam! Bam! And suddenly I was out of breath. I was lightheaded. I got scared, terribly scared, and wanted to get help, but I was so weak I could hardly stand up."

Mr. Insolia was warming up to the subject. He had told the story many times before to other doctors and patients in the hospital, but never did he have an audience like this one. He liked being the center of so much attention. Mr. Insolia paused to look at the students, but Dr. Goldfarb encouraged him to go on with a question.

Every student in the room felt that he already knew what was happening to this man. He was obviously suffering a heart attack or some other cardiac problem.

The fearful pounding accompanied by sudden breathlessness and weakness were the classic symptoms of atrial fibrillation. The atria, two of the heart's four chambers, suddenly start fibrillating—beating wildly but ineffectively. Blood backs up and engorges the lungs.

This almost suffocates the patient, making him feel desperately breathless. Overwhelmed by the resulting drop in blood pressure and inadequate blood circulation, the patient becomes desperately weak. He is terrified by the sudden fatigue, heart pounding, breathlessness. Frequently he is struck by a premonition of impending death.

Going down the checklist of perspectives or dimensions of a symptom for the sake of instruction, Dr. Goldfarb tried to get more details on the chronology and quality of the breathlessness.

"Tell me more about the breathlessness," he said.

"It scared the shit out of me," Mr. Insolia said. "That and the heart pounding. I thought I was going to die."

Mr. Insolia looked awkwardly at two women medical students in the audience, afraid that he might have offended them with the swear word. He hadn't.

"What did you do when this happened?" Dr. Goldfarb asked, trying to find out what helped or aggravated the breathlessness.

Mr. Insolia paused to reconstruct the events in his mind. "I sat down to catch my breath and give my heart a chance to slow down."

"Did it help when you sat down?" Dr. Goldfarb asked. He was thinking of the dynamics of blood flow and oxygenation. Resting would reduce the workload on the impaired heart, which could then pump the blood more effectively. This would improve the oxygenation of the blood and with more oxygen in the circulation the breathlessness would decrease.

"Yeah, it helped a lot when I sat down. At least I think it did," Mr. Insolia said, "because that's when my heart stopped beating crazy and I got my breath back."

"What did you do then?" Dr. Goldfarb asked.

"When I started breathing okay again, I got up and got the next train. I was scared, though. I was afraid that my heart would start racing again. It's really a scary thing."

Dr. Goldfarb said nothing, but he was impressed by the amount of fear Mr. Insolia was describing. Intense fear is common among people suffering atrial fibrillation because the pounding sensation is so strange and strong.

If the breathlessness was a minor thing caused by unaccustomed exertion of emotional problems, the sensation probably wouldn't have been so great as to prompt terror. So the fear itself helped Dr. Goldfarb make the diagnosis.

Mr. Insolia was turning out to be an excellent patient for the student demonstration. Not only did he answer the questions with clarity and brevity, he had a problem that was common, and the symptoms were classic.

Dr. Goldfarb spent almost a half hour questioning Mr. Insolia about the present illness that brought him to the hospital, pursuing every symptom with a batch of questions. Finally he was satisfied that he knew enough and went on to the other four sections of the medical interview—past health, family health, social history, and systems review.

If Dr. Goldfarb had limited his history-taking to discussing the present illness, he would have been led to believe that Mr. Insolia had suddenly been stricken with this problem. From the start, Mr. Insolia had insisted that he "had never been sick a day in his life." But Dr. Goldfarb's continued questioning revealed otherwise. Before Dr. Goldfarb finished the history, it appeared obvious to the students, if not the patient, that this man had been the victim of an insidious disease process that had begun years earlier, when Mr. Insolia thought he was in perfect health.

The first clue that this was a long, ongoing illness was discovered during the part of the interview that dealt with past health. Mr. Insolia was going on at length about how healthy he had been when Dr. Goldfarb suddenly asked him if he ever had swelling around his ankles. Coming out of nowhere, it was a startling question and appeared almost humorously irrelevant.

Mr. Insolia looked at Dr. Goldfarb with surprise, astounded that this physician could have suspected such a trivial thing.

"Yes, I have," Mr. Insolia said, staring at Dr. Goldfarb with uneasy suspicion. "It began a couple of years ago, in the summer. When I came home at night after work I noticed that my ankles were all swollen up like they were going to burst. I got scared and was going to call the doctor, but when I woke up the next morning it wasn't so bad. So I forgot about it."

Several other apparently irrelevant questions turned up interesting clues. Dr. Goldfarb asked Mr. Insolia how many pillows he used at night and discovered that formerly he had used none, but now stacked two under his head.

Mr. Insolia also admitted that he had been having trouble walking up the stairs to his attic workshop, but attributed that to his growing weight and all the cigarettes he had been smoking.

Dr. Goldfarb asked Mr. Insolia if he had ever spit up blood.

Mr. Insolia conceded to this also. He started spitting up blood about a year ago when he started having trouble breathing in bed at night and his ankles started swelling.

Again the cluster of symptoms was classic. Because of the malfunctioning heart, the blood did not move through easily, but backed up into the lungs, building up pressure, which broke small pulmonary vessels that bled.

"What did you do when you started spitting the blood?" Dr. Goldfarb asked.

"I thought I better give up smoking," the man said with an embarrassed smile. The students laughed, but Dr. Goldfarb remained serious.

"You thought you should give up cigarettes!" Dr. Goldfarb said incredulously.

"Yeah," he said.

"You didn't consult a doctor at this point?" he continued.

"I thought it was all from the cigarettes and my weight," Mr. Insolia said, now on the defensive.

"I read about how cigarettes cause shortness of breath and bronchitis, so I thought the bleeding was from that. The ankle swelling I thought was from all the weight I had been putting on."

It took about an hour for Dr. Goldfarb to finish the questioning, but finally it was over and he told Mr. Insolia that he thought he had enough information and asked him if he had anything to add. Mr. Insolia shook his head. The students were then invited to ask questions, but again they had none, so Mr. Insolia was taken back to his room.

Once the patient was gone, Dr. Goldfarb started discussing what had happened.

"I'd like to make one observation before I open this up to discussion," Dr. Goldfarb said. "You have just seen a classic example of patient denial. Most people would have been terrified by the symptoms that this man described, yet he thought it was nothing more than cigarettes and excessive eating. You must keep this in mind when considering what a patient tells you. The denier will minimize his symptoms and incapacity whereas the excessively dependent patient tends to exaggerate every ache and twinge."

After giving the students a chance to diagnose Mr. Insolia's problem incorrectly, Dr. Goldfarb explained that the man had mitral stenosis, probably caused by undiagnosed rheumatic fever as a child.

The mitral valve opening in the man's heart had started to close down to the point where inadequate amounts of blood were being pushed through. The heart was unable to pump the extra blood needed when the man exerted himself. As the condition became worse, fluid began to back up in the lungs and breathlessness occurred.

Dr. Goldfarb finished talking, and after a few seconds of silence a hand was raised at the back of the room. Dr. Goldfarb acknowledged the student.

"Why did you ask him about the pillows?" the student asked.

"Orthopnea," another student said in a stage whisper so Dr. Goldfarb could hear.

Dr. Goldfarb nodded to the whispering student.

"Yes," Dr. Goldfarb said. "Frequently patients with this type of disease will develop breathlessness a few hours after going to bed. Because of the horizontal position, fluids begin accumulating in the lungs. The pillows seem to make the breathing easier."

Another student asked why Dr. Goldfarb asked about the swelling.

Dr. Goldfarb explained that the impaired heart was unable to overcome the effects of gravity, and fluids tended to pool in the lower extremities. That was why the swelling was relieved by a night of rest when the patient was horizontal.

Mr. Insolia was telling the doctors and his friends how his heart disease had started suddenly, with no warning. But to the trained eye of the physician, there were all sorts of warnings. Since the breathlessness dated back almost ten years, Dr. Goldfarb suspected that Mr. Insolia had had heart disease for quite a while. In fact, the process probably started when Mr. Insolia was a boy, stricken by a mild case of rheumatic heart disease he didn't even know he had.

The sun was just beginning to set by the time Helene got home that night. Rather than going right into the house, Helene walked to the city park a block away and sat down on one of the benches. It had been a long day and Helene was tired.

She thought about Mr. Insolia and his heart disease and wondered what the future held for him. It was curious, she thought, that no one had asked how sick he really was, whether the heart disease would progress rapidly and snuff out his life in a few weeks or months or whether the process could be slowed with therapy.

Everyone was concerned with why the doctor asked the questions he did, not with whether the patient would live or die. Helene realized that she couldn't be too critical because she hadn't asked the question either.

Many of the students were like Helene. They had come to medical school determined not to become hard and cynical, concerned only about disease processes and making money, indifferent to the patient as a person.

But, as Helene and the others would learn in the coming months and years, it would be hard always to keep such things in mind. There were too many things to learn, and too little time to do it in, for the students to consider anything much more than the technical matter at hand.

She stood up and walked slowly down the path, hunching her shoulders under her Peruvian poncho to relax the muscles in her tense neck. As she walked, her mind wandered from the park in west Philadelphia to Sarhua and her twin sister. She still thought a lot about Peru, but it wasn't constant the way it was during the first days of medical school. She thought about the natives and the dancing to celebrate important events and the open way everyone related to one another.

It was so different from medical school.

4

The medical school library quickly became a favorite hangout for many of the students whenever they weren't eating, sleeping, or attending classes.

It was a comfortable place, with big easy chairs for reading, study cubicles for those who wanted more privacy, and visual teaching aids to break the monotony of learning from textbooks. But, most important, the library was an escape from the growing sense of loneliness the students were beginning to feel. The students found it a convenient place to drop in on and look for acquaintances or stay awhile to pore over another chapter in Robbins's *Pathologic Basis of Disease,* or Gray's *Anatomy.* Few of the students would dare leave their books for long, but they would chance the brief diversion of talking to fellow classmates as they walked down the long bleak basement corridor that connected the library to the medical college administration building and the Macke lunchroom.

For the more compulsive students afraid to stop working, this corridor and lunchroom is the center of social life for the first semester of medical school. They'd eat snacks and many meals in the Macke, a brightly lit L-shaped room filled with tables, vending machines, and a microwave oven that heated the packaged hot dogs and hamburgers. All other social transactions took place in the corridor outside with its rows of gray steel lockers and long wall of student mailboxes.

In the lockers the students would store the heavy textbooks they brought to school and their anatomy lab coats, smelly from embalming chemicals. And from the mailboxes, assigned to them for their four years at Penn, they would get all communications from the school administration.

☐ ☐ ☐

The library might have been a popular place for many students, but it wasn't for Rikki Lights, who was tending to stay apart from the rest of her class.

Rikki lived in two worlds—one medicine, the other art. The rest of the 159 students in the class could share the medical world with her, but none of them—as far as she could determine so far—were at all interested in her other world. At medical school all the talk was about medicine, but Rikki wanted to talk about poetry and art and music and her feelings.

She had been particularly moved by her experience with her cadaver in the anatomy lab, but she could speak of none of it because her classmates retreated behind the protection of gallows humor. So instead of going to the library or hanging around the Macke room after classes, Rikki would escape to her room or the house of her boyfriend, Ron Gilliam. It was comforting after a day in medical school to go to Ron's place and find him working away at his drums with his brother, James, who played the congas. Ron always greeted her with a smile and stopped for a while to talk to her about her day at school.

And then he'd go back to his drums and she'd go to her books for a few hours. When she got tired of studying, she'd take out her writing book for relaxation and work over a poem she was doing or write another scene for *Ceremony,* a play about a middle class black woman. After a few hours of writing she'd go back to the medical books.

Rikki's art wasn't the only thing that set her apart from the rest of her class. There was also her sex and race. Though it was true that women and minority students were entering medical schools in unprecedented numbers, medicine still was essentially a white and male world and Rikki was very much aware of this.

When she felt the pinch of actual or imagined prejudice in medical school, however, she wasn't sure whether it was her being black, a woman, or both that was to blame. Being sensitive, Rikki may have been seeing more prejudice than actually existed, but she didn't think so.

One day in the Macke room, a man she had met in class asked her what it was like to be a black in a mostly white world. At first she was suspicious, but then she decided to take a chance and reveal herself.

The prejudice strikes deep, she said, and makes its victims question the most basic aspects of their worth, even the way they look as human beings.

"The culture dictated that I not consider myself attractive," Rikki said, sipping coffee out of a paper cup from one of the vending machines. "I'm not white. And my nose isn't straight. And my hair is not straight. And my lips are not small. People would look at me and say 'Rikki Lights is not at all attractive. She's ugly.' That's what society said of me. If you don't look Caucasian, you were not attractive.

"So I had to come to terms with how I looked and with my standards of beauty. 'What the heck,' I said to myself, 'I don't see anything ugly about me. There are things about my face that are unique. Why can't I groove on that?'

"The people who think I'm not attractive because I'm not Caucasian are the same people who think that there's nothing special about me because I'm black and female and in medicine. And medicine is an all-white and all-male field. If they had their way, that's the way it would remain."

The man said he understood, but Rikki didn't think he did. She wondered if she should have spoken so openly to him. Rikki was becoming very wary, prompted partly by an unpleasant experience during her first month at Penn.

It was a day on which Rikki had come to class in a particularly casual style of dress. She never wore girdles and on this day wasn't even wearing a bra. While in pathology class, bent over a microscope studying blood cells, a white classmate came over to her. He was one of the younger boys in the class.

Bending down to Rikki and bringing his lips close to her ear, he whispered: "I can tell you don't have a bra on."

Rikki's body tensed. Snapping her face to the right, she saw this grinning face next to hers.

"You know how I can tell?" he said, still grinning and keeping his face close to hers.

"No," Rikki said, glowering at the youth. "How can you tell?"

"Because I can see your tits moving up and down under your sweater," he said, giggling.

Rikki was still mad when she got to Ron's place that night. "You know what happened to me in pathology?" she said, and Ron stopped practicing to hear the story.

When she was through, he just shook his head. He could not believe that in only four years this youth would be a physician.

The next day Rikki bought the first girdle she had owned in years. It was an extreme thing for a young woman to do in the age of free-style dress and the women's movement, but under the circumstances Rikki was taking no chances.

The contrast between the cold world of medicine and the warm and supporting world of art was drawing Rikki even closer to Ron.

Every time she was rebuffed in medical school or felt isolated or different from all the rest of the students, Rikki could turn to Ron and find someone she could identify with.

Ron could understand Rikki's need to write and express herself artistically even if it meant that some time would be taken away from her medical books.

He could understand and appreciate the way she expressed herself with forceful language and emotional enthusiasm even though it might not be the professional way, which demanded detachment if not aloofness.

Rikki's relationship with Ron, which had begun a year earlier when she met him at a jazz concert, was growing deeper. It didn't matter so much that her classmates weren't interested in the same things that she was.

□ □ □

Ron was a cheerful, good-looking man with the slender wiry build of someone who used his body vigorously, which he did for hours while playing the drums. Working the big drum and cymbals with his legs and the smaller drums with his arms was physically demanding.

Ron was about the same age as most of the students in Rikki's class, but he seemed much more mature. A lifetime of hard work to support himself and start a career in the competitive world of music had made Ron wise about many things that the students, who had never left the sheltered environment of the campus, were still naïve about.

In recent months Ron had been growing tired much more quickly than before. And his headaches were getting worse, so much so that he would roll about in bed, clasping his hands to his head, moaning: "Oh, my head, my head, my head."

The headaches had begun a year earlier, when Rikki was still at Bryn Mawr College. She had attributed them to the tensions of Ron's demanding life. But Rikki became increasingly concerned as the headaches persisted.

She became terrified in medical school when she started pathology class and read about the terrible things that could cause headaches. The most fearful possibility was a brain tumor, but Ron had none of the associated neurologic symptoms, such as paralysis or loss of mental acuity.

Then Rikki began to study high blood pressure, in particular renal hypertension, which is high blood pressure associated with kidney trouble. Poring over the big purple textbook—Robbins's *Pathologic Basis of Disease*—Rikki read and reread the section on kidney disease. It was here that she first came upon the term *lipoid nephrosis,* a kidney problem that usually affected children but in most cases eventually disappeared without causing any lasting trouble.

The legs of children with this problem would swell up as the tissue filled with fluids backed up behind the malfunctioning kidneys. The usual treatment was to give corticosteroid drugs, prednisone in particular. It was a good sign if the patient responded to the prednisone because this usually meant that there would be no lasting kidney damage. But Rikki also read that in a few situations the kidney problems reappeared in adulthood, leading to high blood pressure, headaches, vomiting, weakness, and often death.

Renal hypertension. The two words assumed menacing proportions for Rikki. Ron would be in serious trouble if his headaches were a symptom of renal hypertension. Rikki chided herself for being a hysterical medical student. All medical students become hypochondriacs at one time or another during their four years of study. They spend so much time reading about the symptoms of lethal diseases that after a while they begin to detect comparable aches and pains in themselves or people close to them and they begin worrying about imminent death.

At first Rikki tried to dismiss her fears, but finally she gave in and started asking Ron questions about his medical history. Ron was amused by Rikki's concern, but he conceded that he did have edema as a child. His legs would swell up so big that he'd have to stay home, he said.

"Did you go to the doctor?" Rikki asked. "Did they give you anything for it?"

Yes, he did go to the doctors and they did give him a drug that worked. It was prednisone. He did have kidney disease as a child.

All at once Rikki's darkest fears were realized. But could it be possible, Rikki asked herself, that the first diagnosis of her career was correct, that she had identified a comparatively unusual disease on the basis of an incomplete medical history and a single symptom as common as a headache? She didn't even know for certain that Ron had high blood pressure. Maybe the headaches were associated with tension and had nothing to do with high blood pressure or kidney disease or any other lethal problem.

But Rikki was still frightened enough to insist that Ron see a doctor. At first he refused, but he quickly changed his mind when she started talking about brain tumors.

Ron was in a good mood when he came back from the clinic. He didn't have a brain tumor, he told Rikki with obvious relief. It was only high blood pressure, he said.

A few days later Rikki called the office of Dr. Anna-Marie Chirico, a highly respected internist at HUP (the Hospital of the University of Pennsylvania).

"I would like to make an appointment for a very dear friend of mine," she told the appointment secretary. "It's very important that Dr. Chirico see him right away. I'm a medical student and I think that my friend has renal hypertension."

5

As the days turned into weeks and the weeks became months, the students in the class of '78 began to fall into the routine of medical school.

A hurried breakfast at the big wood tables in the Stouffers Triangle restaurant, a race down Hamilton Walk under branches that were becoming bare, and another morning of lectures in pathology or dissection in anatomy.

More classes in the afternoon, a little bit of socializing over dinner, and then back to the library or room or apartment or commune for three or four hours of solitary book work.

One twenty-year-old student from the Midwest found she had become a virtual hermit. Each night she would go to her fifth-floor apartment in the Graduate Towers, a modern but sterile high-rise on the Penn campus, sit down at her desk at the window, and stay there until 12:30, studying textbooks too large to put comfortably in her lap. Her only distraction during these vigils was the lonely view of another student sitting in front of his window in the Graduate Towers' wing opposite her, studying late into the night.

She was trapped by her loneliness. But Ronald Cargill, whose first year in medical school was being paid for by the Black Muslims, was purposely isolating himself from most of the class. He had learned to be a loner in the ghettos of Harlem and Camden, New Jersey, and now he was using the protection of distance in the foreign environment of medical school.

A small incident during one of the first lectures had put Ron on guard. He was sitting in one of the crowded lectures halls when a white student next to him crossed his legs and brushed Ron's papers with his foot.

"Hey watch that!" Ron said to the student, who gave him first a dirty look and then smart talk that Ron never would have tolerated in the ghetto.

"What are you yelling at me for?" the student said, sneering at Ron. "What can I do? It's cramped in here and I need room, too."

The next day Ron arrived at school wearing one of his broad-brimmed hats. Looking more like an old-time Chicago hood than a medical student, Ron was now set apart from all the other students. The outlandish hat had an intimidating quality because the broad brim shielded Ron's eyes, virtually cutting off all contact between him and those around him. It was most important to establish that he was different and not someone to be confronted or disturbed.

Ron and the other students were beginning to discover that the medical school—nestled behind the Spruce Street dormitories on the Penn campus—was becoming family, community, and subculture to them. They had entered a superspecialized insular world, into which even television and newspapers rarely intruded.

For many the only remaining links with the outside world were weekend trips back home or visits from boyfriends or girl friends. The old friends were allowed to intrude only briefly, however—a few hours after anatomy on Saturday and a fleeting Sunday. Then the grind would start up again Monday morning, with those who played too much feeling a guilt that would keep them at their books the next weekend.

If it was true, as some claimed, that the typical physician was socially isolated and unable to emphathize with nonphysicians, then perhaps the process of alienation was already beginning for some of the students.

□ □ □

The students might have been isolating themselves from the rest of the world so that they could study but, as they were finding out in the hospitals, the rest of the world was tending to isolate them also, putting them on pedestals because they were on their way to becoming physicians.

Anxious patients, confronting pain, death, or sickness, have a vested interest in believing in their physicians and attributing to them powers that tend to elevate and separate them. The students had been warned about this by Dr. Martin T. Orne, an eloquent psychiatry professor who held his audiences spellbound with his dry wit.

"The range of things a patient will do in front of a doctor is amazing," Dr. Orne said during one lecture, twirling a cigar he never lit.

"He does it not because of your sterling character but because of the relationship. You'll wear a white coat and your patient will expect a lot from you even though you don't know a hell of a lot more than you did a couple of weeks ago when you didn't wear a white coat.

"Patients have a vested interest in believing in their doctor," Dr. Orne continued. "You have to mess up very badly to lose that trust. I've interviewed a lot of people the night before they went to surgery and I have yet to meet one person who didn't think that his surgeon was the best one in the world. Can you imagine lying there in bed thinking that the doctor who will be operating on you tomorrow is a bum?"

The specialized knowledge the students were acquiring was also beginning to separate them from nonmedical people. The magic and uniqueness of human life was being stripped away and replaced by rational, frequently mechanistic, concepts. The human heart had become a bundle of pulsating cardiac cells. The brain was composed of nothing more than neurons that transmitted electrical signals. And the human body, violated by scalpel with viscera exposed, was reduced to an insignificance that left the medical students momentarily stunned.

But just as this knowledge tainted any poetic reverence for human life, it also would promote, eventually, a sense of wonder for the biologic complexities that made life possible.

Dr. David D. Rowlands, Jr., chairman of the pathology department, and Dr. Leonard Berwick exposed the students to this wonder with their descriptions of the amazing processes the body used to protect itself from disease.

Writing each new term or technical word on the blackboard to help the students learn the foreign language they as physicians must eventually speak, Drs. Rowland and Berwick led the students through the maze of biochemical reactions that begin the moment a threatening foreign substance enters the body and ends weeks or months later with the frail balance of health usually restored.

It was a dramatic story of thousands of battles being waged among millions of cells. It was a story about antibodies attacking antigens, about cells living and cells dying. But it was a drama often lost in the mass of material that had to be absorbed.

It wasn't drama that the students were seeing, but rather the confusing technicalities of biology and biochemistry. And so much had to be remembered—sequence of events, cluster of facts, thousands of words.

The bone marrow produced the lymphocytes that produced the antibodies that reacted with the antigens that lie somewhere on the pathogens.

The visible signs of inflammation were redness, swelling, heat, and pain. The process was contraction, dilation, margination, and emigration.

And the words—histamine, bradykinin, serotonin.

It would be months, maybe years, before the wonder would become apparent. Undergraduate biology had a poetic simplicity by comparison. A white cell was a white cell was a white cell. Now a white cell was a neutrophil, an eosinophil, and a basophil.

Perhaps it could all be remembered with a few more hours of study. But there was never enough time because tomorrow was anatomy. The anatomical words were in Latin—coxa, nates, femur, genu. That meant hip, buttock, thigh, knee. Eighty words to remember this night plus forty from last week when the student fell behind.

And always there were the questions that seemed to pop up while shaving or waiting for the elevator or watching clouds floating by in the sky.

What about the thoracic wall and mediastinum?

Gray's *Anatomy,* that hideous text, would explain:

The external intercostal muscles are attached to the lower margins of each of the first eleven ribs. Their fibers pass downward and forward to the upper margin of the rib below. The lower seven muscles are intimately connected with the external oblique.

Over and over the students would reread these passages, trying to remember it all, trying to master it.

"The lower seven muscles are intimately connected with the external oblique."

And their tired minds would wander, and silly thoughts would be pondered.

How could anything be intimate with an external oblique?

And so it went. Words. Terms. Verbal descriptions that inadequately portrayed three-dimensional relationships. It was a difficult world, a frightening world. No matter how easy the professors tried to make it, it was always difficult.

Going to school had come to be a tightrope walk over a bottomless chasm. The student had to pay very careful attention and never lose his place because he knew if he did—even for a second—that he would fall into that chasm.

6

Most of the students left Philadelphia for the Thanksgiving holidays and spent the long weekend with their families and friends. Though they had been gone less than three months, things seemed different when they got back home. They didn't know whether it was their imagination or something real, but it felt like they were being treated with a little more respect, as though their opinions mattered more. A few of the students were even asked for advice on medical problems by friends who assumed that they had gained special insight about such things during their brief time in medical school.

Some students used the few days away from school as an opportunity to forget medicine and revisit a wider world. It was good to talk about the politics in the newspapers again and about art and literature.

It was a luxury to lie in bed and contemplate shadows on the wall from the morning sun or listen to the noise of breakfast being made in the kitchen, knowing that there was no need to get up right away, knowing that this day at least would not have to start at the cadaver table.

The holidays were disappointing, however, for some parents who were unable to find out how their children liked medical school. It is difficult for a student to tell parents who are working hard to pay the high tuition and who had dreamed so long about one's becoming a physician that medical school is a disappointment.

How could you tell your parents that you hate medical school because the work is overwhelming and the other students are so competitive and it's not intellectually exciting and everything on television and in the movies about doctors is a lot of bunk? But mostly how could you tell your parents that you aren't sure you want to become a doctor.

So instead the student says nothing. And his parents are allowed to believe they are doing so much for him.

□ □ □

The students returned to school from Thanksgiving holidays with renewed energy to finish out the first semester. Final exams were only a month away. The big day was December 16. That was when the first of the five final exams would be given. And then there would be another exam every day until Decemeber 20, when it would all be over and the students could start a twenty-three-day vacation.

As December 16 approached, the mood in medical school became progressively more tense because the pressures of studying were increasing. The students tended to be more brusque and passed each other in the halls without pausing for conversation.

In the Macke vending machine room students read books instead of talking as they ate their microwave-heated sandwiches. And the social life —severely restricted at best of times—had become nonexistent.

Many students came to the anatomy lab late at night to probe their cadavers one more time, looking for the muscle or artery they might be asked to identify during the anatomy test.

The growing anxiety among the students as finals week approached could best be seen in the anatomy laboratory, where they rushed from cadaver to cadaver comparing the appearances of various anatomical structures.

"I just want to go to the movies when this is all over," one student told a friend, a little nervous that she was talking instead of working on her nearby cadaver.

"I'm going to go to New York for a week and see movies three times a day. Oh, I'll be so glad when this is all over. Oh, I'll be so glad," she repeated to herself as she and her friend returned to their illustrated anatomy books, incongruously propped up on music stands next to the cadavers so that the students could identify the parts they were dissecting.

Suddenly, a dozen students rushed to one of the tables where white-haired Professor Robert J. Johnson had started to give a special demonstration, using a new specimen that had been sliced into small sections to show interior parts. The students crowded close to the table and peered over the shoulders of those in front. Some of the smaller ones stood on stools to get a view.

Though the students had other courses, anatomy was without question the one that was getting top priority for study. There were many reasons, the principal one being the fearful thought of spending another semester repeating the tedious task of dissecting a body and learning all of the parts again.

Anatomy on this level was neither intellectually demanding nor satisfying, but it took a lot of time and a good memory to get the information in hand long enough to repeat it back during exams.

No one could say how many parts went to make up the human body because it depended on how precise one wanted to be in the description. But a good anatomist had a couple of thousand structures delineated in his mind.

These students had about a thousand nerves, muscles, arteries, bones, and other items to worry about—or at least that was how many were included in the class notes given to them at the start of the year.

The special demonstration over, twenty-one-year-old Walter Tsou returned to his table and carefully consulted his anatomical atlas on its music stand. "It's like taking the first hundred pages of the Philadelphia telephone book and deciding to memorize them," he said, shaking his head and picking up an anatomy probe.

"Are you worried about the exam?" someone asked him with mock shock.

"I'm not uptight about it," he said.

"You're not?" shot back Barbara Turner, who was one of the six-member dissecting team at Walter's table. "You must have changed a lot since last week."

"I've been here late the last few days," he replied.

One student had stayed in the lab until 3:00 A.M. He worked on the cadaver by himself in the silent and empty room, checking out various structures against the descriptions and sketches in his anatomy book, and then returned the next morning at 7:00 A.M.

During orientation week in September, a lot of students laughed when anatomy professor Jean Piatt told them that the labs would be kept open twenty-four hours a day so they could dissect whenever they wanted.

At the time, it sounded like a ludicrous, even slightly macabre, offer. But it didn't seem that way the week before final exams.

□ □ □

The prodding anxiety that kept students at their books and in the anatomy lab late into the night was being joined by a growing hostility toward the school. The griping could be heard in the Macke room from students hunched closely together over the tables so that professors who happened into the room would not hear.

"What gripes me," one student said to two classmates, "is that they treat us with the same formality and distance that the doctors treat patients. You wouldn't think of calling any of them by their first names."

The two other heads nodded in thoughtful agreement. "Yeah," one of the other students said. "It's not like undergrad. I remember this one art professor. Everyone called him Al. After classes we'd go out drinking beer together. Or in the summer, when it was a beautiful day, he'd rush into class and take us all out to the park where we'd eat bread and cheese and sketch and talk. Could you imagine one of them running into anatomy lab, saying it's too beautiful a day to stay there and let's all go out for cheese and bread under the trees?" Everyone laughed at the impossible scene. Then they got up and went back to the library or anatomy laboratory.

Two other students had found privacy in the rear row of one of the empty lecture halls where they nibbled on sandwiches together. They knew each other from undergraduate school at Penn and had become fairly close friends.

After a long silence, one of them said:

"You know, I've been trying to deny this ever since we started classes here, but I can't deny it any longer." He didn't look at his friend as he spoke, but instead looked down the empty rows of seats that led to the speaker's pit, where a few months earlier Dean Stemmler had welcomed them to medical school.

"You can't deny what?" his friend finally said.

"I made a mistake coming to medical school," he said thoughtfully. "It was all a mistake. I'm no doctor. I can't remember all this shit. I'm no doctor. You know what I mean?"

His friend looked at him with neither amusement nor surprise. He took another bite of his sandwich, nodded, and his friend sighed.

Another student sat by herself in one of the study cubicles in the library. In a few minutes she would go back to the anatomy laboratory, but first she wanted to read up more in pathology because she felt she had been neglecting it.

After several minutes, she realized that the words she was seeing in the book had nothing to do with her thoughts. She kept thinking back to the Thanksgiving holidays and her college friends who were just beginning their careers and furnishing their homes with their first paychecks.

They had all been filled with an excitement that she seemed to have lost over the past few months. She gave up trying to read Robbins, snapped off the cubicle light, and lay her head on the purple textbook. No one could tell how badly she was feeling because she didn't sob. And in the darkness of the cubicle no one could see the tears sliding down her cheeks.

□ □ □

The week before the final exams of the first semester has always been a period of self-doubt, anger, and sadness for medical students. That's because the exams constitute the first acute stress the students have met since entering medical school. All the forced study preceding the exams makes them aware of the long hours and tedious work that a medical career demands.

Dean Stemmler could sense the tense atmosphere as he walked through the halls and past the labs where the students worked. He knew from his experience with many other first semesters that the mood would be different next term. The students would be calmer and more relaxed because they wouldn't be under the same kind of heat.

Dr. Piatt could never understand why the students got so worked up, especially in his anatomy course. "It's practically impossible for them to flunk out," he said, surveying the students working over the cadavers in the brightly lit room. "I just can't understand why they're so worried about this course, because you don't need any background for anatomy. You could teach a bright twelve-year-old student all of this."

Dr. Piatt was right. Failures didn't occur that often, though it was true that there were more failures in anatomy than in any other of the classes the first-year students took.

But even if a student did fail anatomy, he could take a month-long, makeup course in the summer and take another test before starting his second year. Failing this, he would then take the course over again. One student repeated the course three times before squeezing past.

The students in the class of '78 were nervous even though they also knew how well the students who preceded them—the students in the class of '77—had done on these very same tests only a year earlier.

Only four of them failed anatomy, three failed physiology and two flunked pathology. No one failed histology. It looked even better from an overall point of view. Only two students from the previous class had to take leaves of absences for psychiatric or academic reasons and only two students in the class of '78 were in similar troubles.

Most of the students were aware of the optimistic statistics, but still they worked five or six hours a night and all day and night on weekends.

There were many reasons why they worked so hard, even though the overwhelming evidence indicated that there was nothing to worry about. The most obvious explanation was that the highly selective admissions policies of medical schools, which accept only one of three applicants, screen out the more casual and let in only the hard workers.

Medical students respond to stress by working even harder. If they let stress or hard work bother them, they wouldn't have come as far as they had. The dean felt that it was partly a trait retained from the highly competitive world of the pre-med student, who is working against odds to get into any medical school, let alone a good one.

"Students have always overworked in the first semester," Dean Stemmler said, "because they don't know what is expected of them. They refuse to believe what we told them—that we are not trying to screen them out. They won't believe that until they have had a chance to prove it out for themselves."

□ □ □

The last few days and nights before the start of final exam week were awful. The hour of the day or night had little meaning because the only important thing was the number of study hours remaining before December 16.

It didn't matter whether it was 10:00 in the morning or 10:00 at night. The weather was immaterial. Rain, snow, or sunlight—it made no difference because everything that mattered was inside the buildings, inside the books, hopefully inside the minds.

Even years later, when these students were successful doctors in practice for themselves, they would remember the nights before finals because the nights were the worst.

At night, many of the students preferred to work in the library or some other hideaway on campus rather than being entombed in their rabbit warren apartments in Graduate Towers. They said it was because they were afraid of being seduced by the comfort of a nearby bed or stereo set, but more basic psychic needs were at work.

There was comfort working near some fellow sufferer even if there was no communication. It prevented the students from hallucinating that they were the last people on earth, hidden and forgotten, behind a plywood door, tormented by too much work and not enough time.

The mood at night in medical school was decidedly different from that of the daytime. The night sounds and the night people take over.

Steam hissed through overhead pipes in now silent halls. Way down at the end, past the mailboxes and steel lockers that are closed and silent, a first-year student walked out of the brightly lit vending machine room and then disappeared down another hall.

The little socializing that was going on during that week seemed to take place in this grim hallway with its harsh lighting. It almost became the equivalent of a promenade deck on a cruise liner, with students chatting briefly on their way from the library to the Macke room or the anatomy lab in yet another connecting building.

The modern decor of the library was more homey than the rest of the building at night because of the easy chairs and carpets. Most of the seats were filled with students reading silently. Some yawned because it was late at night and it had been a tiring day. Others sat in front of color teaching television sets, looking at oddly silent pictures and listening to words over headphones.

Outside the library and down the promenade hallway leading to the vending machine room a group of students argued briefly over whether this would be the worst week of their careers as physicians.

"No, no," said one woman medical student. "The first week of internship will be the worst week because you're on your own and responsible for making important decisions."

"Yes, that may be true," said another medical student with a day's growth of beard that made his face look dirty, "but you don't have to worry about flunking out."

They talked a bit more and then went in different directions. At the other end of the hallway, a university security guard walked down a deserted hall with a night-watch clock strapped around his neck, checking locked doors. A cleaning man swept the sloping floors of Lecture Room D.

And the first-year students all studied for the final exams that they were about to begin.

7

Bundled against a driving rain on a morning so dark that some street lights were still on, the students started arriving for their first final exam at 8:30, a half hour before the test was to begin.

Crowding in the hallway outside of the Macke room, they crammed soggy coats and books into the gray steel lockers. There seemed to be more talking and joking than usual, a hedge against tension and fatigue.

"How's it going?" someone asked Jim Nestor.

"It's a bummer," he said, pushing through the door into Lecture Room B, one of the two where the exam would be given. They were using two rooms because seats were so jammed together in the lecture halls that it would be difficult to prevent cheating.

Rikki Lights arrived, but she was more preoccupied with Ron than the exam she was about to take. Ron had been admitted to the HUP the night before on Dr. Chirico's service. Dr. Chirico wanted to determine the cause of Ron's high blood pressure, and a battery of tests would be needed to check on Ron's kidneys as well as other things.

Rikki was still convinced that her original diagnosis of renal hypertension was right, but she was hoping desperately that she was wrong. Ron could sense her concern, even though Rikki tried to hide it behind her anxiety over the final exams. But instead of talking about Ron's impending hospitalization, Ron and Rikki had talked about the exams, with Ron assuring her that she would do just fine.

Steve Levine arrived in Lecture Room B in generally good spirits, though he looked gaunt and had several days' growth of beard on his normally clean-shaven face. For almost a week Steve had been sick with a viral infection so debilitating that the infirmary tried to keep him overnight, but he refused. He wanted to stay home and study. He did stay home, but was just too sick to study.

The exam started a few minutes late with a humorless exam proctor telling the students that the test was not on the honor system, and that they would be watched. Everyone laughed.

The test involved one hundred multiple-choice questions, so long and complicated in their formulation that the exam ran to seventeen pages and would require three hours to complete.

The proctors distributed the mimeographed tests, working from the front to the back of the roomful of buzzing students. A wake of silence followed the physiology exam papers up the rows of seats as the students started reading the questions. Soon everyone had the test and the room was silent.

Physiology is the study of normal living function, as opposed to pathology, which is the study of disease. It is a comparatively precise area of medicine, requiring an understanding of complicated natural functions, on both a biochemical and a mechanical level.

As the test progressed, the lecture halls were unusually quiet with little coughing or paper rustling. The students sat for many minutes staring down at the test paper with their pens and pencils held up.

Gradually they would eliminate the alternative answers in their minds until only one of the multiple choice alternatives remained. They would then lower their pens, make quick circles around the selected answers, and move on to the next question.

The only sound was the rain outside and the roar of an unseen jet overhead.

Katharine Treadway left the room for a drink of water, staring down at the floor all the way down the hall and back.

"How's it going?" she was asked.

"I don't know," she said. "It certainly is harder than the midterms." Kate was one of the most academically gifted students in the class of '78 and in four years would graduate at the top of her class.

The proctor got up and updated the time written on the blackboard to guide the students. He had just marked 10:55 when William Warwick, the son and grandson of doctors, became the first to complete the test, an hour and forty-five minutes after it had begun, and an hour and fifteen minutes before the time would be up.

"It was like they told us," he said, bounding down the hall to the Macke room for something to eat. "You don't have to memorize a lot of little things."

For a while Bill sat by himself in the empty Macke room, drinking coffee from a paper cup and nibbling on a sandwich that he had brought with him in a brown paper bag. But soon the vending machine room began to fill with students who had completed the test before the allotted three hours.

"I'm pretty certain of seventy-five of the questions," one student said.

Another said that he didn't think he did anywhere near that well. Then, with resignation, he added, "They say the first year isn't that important anyhow."

Kate Treadway came in, obviously tired, still a little tense. She had lost eight pounds since medical school started and she wasn't overweight then.

"I guess I did about medium," she said.

The exam was supposed to end at noon, but when twelve o'clock arrived there were still thirty to forty students in the exam rooms. They could take an extra hour if they wanted, though this fact would be noted on the paper, the proctor said.

At 12:15 an obviously bushed student came out, smiled at a friend, and philosophized: "Oh, well, they say it's a guessing game."

The last student to finish the exam came out of Lecture Room B at a little past 1:00 P.M., shaking his head.

"That was unbelievable," he said. "That was really bad. That was a rough exam. I mean, that was not an easy test."

He kept saying the same thing in different ways over and over as he walked down the hall.

The Macke room was filled with students now. So much excess energy was being released that it was hard for people to hear each other above the din. Based on snatches of a dozen different conversations, the consensus seemed to be that the test was very difficult, but most students thought they had passed. A good mark was another question. The students couldn't be completely frank with each other about their worry because Penn was on a pass/fail system with no numerical grades. To complain about a passing grade no matter what it was would be to suggest a desire for an "honors" grade. Admitting such a competitive streak was not the thing to do in this class.

For about an hour, the students talked excitedly in the vending machine room. And then they started dispersing. Some went home for a nap. Many went to the library to study for the next exams.

It was still raining hard outside and the sidewalk glistened with rain.

□ □ □

The twenty-eight cadavers were lined up in rows on the anatomy laboratory tables and each one was tagged with numbered labels. It looked like a rummage sale of bodies. But this was the tag quiz, or "musical bodies," as some of the students called it.

When the first-year students first heard about it from students in the classes ahead of them, they thought it was a joke, but it wasn't. The test consisted of parading down rows of cadavers and identifying the nerves, arteries, muscles, and organs tagged with the numbered labels.

Because there weren't enough bodies to go around, the class was broken into three sections, which took the exam at ninety-minute intervals.

To prevent the chaos of an Easter egg hunt, the students would advance in orderly fashion from body to body in time to a buzzer sounded at sixty-second intervals. They'd examine the part of the body that was tagged, write the name of the part next to the corresponding number on their exam papers, and then wait for the next buzz. When it sounded, they'd move quickly on to the next body down the line, repeating the process every minute until fifty parts had been identified. The students could not tarry or else they would be overtaken by those advancing from the preceding corpse.

Getting the students' attention, Dr. Piatt explained the rules of the test, asked if there were any questions, and then told them to begin.

The sudents quickly examined the tagged parts at the tables they stood at, made the appropriate notation, and then rushed on to the next table when the buzzer sounded. They ran fast, even though the next table was only a few feet away, almost as grown-ups do in the games they play on daytime television.

Steve Levine, still sick from the viral infection, looked terrible as he dragged himself from body to body. His growth of beard was heavier than the day before and he still had a fever and felt bad. He couldn't have become sick at a worse time. After the quiz, he finally gave up and made arrangements to take his other tests after he got back from vacation.

Finally the buzzer sounded for the fiftieth and last time; the students made the final notation in their test booklet and waited to be dismissed. Then the laughing and joking began because the anatomy test everyone was dreading was over and it had been much easier than they had thought it would be. This suggested to the students that the written part of the anatomy test to be given the next day would also be easy.

Dr. Piatt dismissed the students and the first section went laughing and yelling out the swinging doors, giving the thumbs up sign to the classmates in section two, waiting in the hallway to begin their test.

□ □ □

The written part of the anatomy test turned out to be frighteningly more difficult than anyone thought it would be, especially after the easy tag quiz the day before. It was bad. And for the first time since finals began, students began to talk in terms of possibly failing.

One student came out of Lecture Room B, hunched up his shoulders in a shiver, and sighed. Others followed him out, singly and in pairs. There was no laughing, hardly any talking, only the hushed exchange of concern between worried students.

Twenty-four hours later, with the completion of the pathology exam, the mood in the hallways was completely different. Even before the exam was half over, the students knew everything would be all right. They smiled when they came out of the exam room for a break and they joked in the hallway afterward.

Now, students began to talk about what they'd be doing on their twenty-three-day vacation, which would begin the moment they finished the physiology exam on Friday, now less than a day away.

Rikki finished the exam in good time, packed up her books and pads and walked out on to Hamilton Walk. It was a gray, wet, depressing day.

Shivering from the cold, she walked down the path, entered the Thirty-sixth Street entrance of the HUP and made her way through the maze of interconnected buildings to the Ravdin wing where Ron was.

The twenty-six-year-old musician was drumming away on a drumming practice pad when Rikki arrived. Dressed in a T-shirt and hospital pajama pants, he looked in good shape, though his face appeared a little puffy from edema. He smiled when Rikki entered, but kept working the practice pads.

"Pathology was all right," Rikki said, plumping down on Ron's unused bed.

Ron stopped for a moment and nodded.

"I told you you would do good." Then he started again.

"Get any results back?" she asked.

Ron shook his head. "And as far as I'm concerned no news is good news." Rikki smiled.

The two young people were just beginning to move with their careers— Ron with his music and Rikki with her writing and medicine. It was such an exciting time for the two of them because all of the work they had been doing separately and together was about to pay off.

But now everything was turned upside down.

The test results finally came back and Rikki was right. Ron had renal hypertension. His kidneys were dying. In a little while, they would stop producing urine completely and a long chain of grim events would begin for Ron—kidney dialysis, a kidney transplant that wouldn't work, and then the irrevocable, lifetime sentence of being attached to a machine three times a week to keep the poisons in his body from killing him.

But Rikki and Ron didn't talk about the grim things that possibly lay ahead of them. Instead he talked about her final exams and she talked about his practicing and possible gigs. They both talked about how it was such a gray, depressing day and so close to Christmas.

□ □ □

The cork exploded out of the champagne bottle with a pop, hit the ceiling of the Macke, and ricocheted, almost hitting a student who was about to make a pass with a football. Everyone laughed, and the champagne flowed. Final exams were over.

As predicted, histology, the study of cells and the way they work, was the easiest of the five exams taken all week. The exam was supposed to take three hours, but many students were done by 10:00 A.M.—after only one hour—and it was only 11:15 when the champagne was opened.

Matt Lotysh, who finally arranged at the last moment to raise the fare for a trip back to California, came bounding down the hall with a camera to take pictures of the school.

"I get on a plane at eleven thirty tonight," he said, "and by four thirty tomorrow morning I'll be in San Francisco. Marge has made reservations for dinner at dawn—you can do that in San Francisco—and by Sunday I'll be scuba diving. And it's going to be warm. And I'm just going to let my mind be free."

A woman student came into the Macke and hugged the first person she ran into. More champagne was poured. And for the first time all year, some students arrived wearing suits and ties, presumably leaving the campus for more civilized environs.

Upstairs on the first-floor of the Johnson Pavilion, where the exams were still being given, the hallway had been turned into a small cocktail lounge by one of the women students who had brought some of the bubbly wine for her fellow students and her husband.

The husband sat up on a desk in the hall with a funny stocking cap on his head, while their two-year-old daughter played with an empty bottle.

He had brought the child up from Washington, where they lived, to celebrate the end of tests for her mother. For the last sixteen weeks, he had worked and taken care of the girl while his wife went to school, the three commuting on weekends to get together. Now they could live like a normal family for twenty-three days.

Down the hall within painful earshot of the impromptu party, four or five students still bent over their exam papers finishing the nine essay questions and trying to ignore the laughing and joking.

With the exception of physiology, no grades would be available until the students returned from vacation in January, but most knew already whether they had passed or failed.

A student came bounding down the hall with a test paper in hand. Contriving to boast as modestly as possible, he said to a classmate: "Only nine wrong. They must have made a mistake."

"How'd you get your marks on today's test so fast?" someone else asked.

"This is physiology. Remember physiology. The test we took a life-time ago last Monday. The grades are in. They must have made a mistake because I got only nine wrong."

"You got honors," another student said, seeing the word written clearly on top of the paper.

"No kidding," he replied, trying to pretend surprise. "I won't accept it."

Though the mood was primarily a happy one, a hint of sadness hid among the laughter and champagne. For sixteen weeks the students had been brought together as a cohesive whole, welded together by the demands of their common education.

But those demands were lifted now, at least temporarily, and the community of students was breaking up, each student en route to distant points and people and things that had nothing to do with their friends and second life in the medical school.

For three weeks the subculture would no longer exist.

Now that the finals were all over, the tension and anxiety that had kept these students going began to fade, and exhaustion began to set in. Many students said they would celebrate a little later. For the present all they wanted was a bed and a peaceful sleep, knowing that tomorrow would bring no more tests.

It was 12:30 by the time the last student walked out of the medical school building into the bright, crisp December afternoon. The trees on Hamilton Walk were bare now. The art students, who in the warmth of September sat in the grass sketching the old medical school building, were gone now. And the people hurried by because it was too cool to dally in long conversation.

The first semester was over.

8

The students returned from Christmas vacation refreshed and relaxed, unaware that the most difficult period of their schooling was over—only four months after they'd started.

The first semester at Penn was like a hazing to get into a fraternity or the initiation rites of a primitive tribe. The curriculum committee hadn't planned it that way. It was just that a medical student had to master an immense amount of basic information before he could begin to learn how to become a doctor.

At Penn most of this information was given in a concentrated dose during the first year, and it just happened that the first half of the first year was much more difficult than the second half.

The second semester had only thirty-one hours of class and lab work each week as compared to thirty-eight hours during the first semester. There would be only two major science courses—neurobiology and biochemistry—this term as compared to three heavy classes last year.

Neurobiology, which met three hours a day, three days a week, would be a demanding course. It was a combination lecture and lab course in which the students probed the human brain and studied the diverse functions of the nervous system. The course was heavy with philosophical and clinical implications.

The biochemistry course met four hours a day on Mondays, Wednesdays, and Fridays. Here the students would study the myriad of biochemical reactions that are continually going on in living organisms.

Two other courses during the second semester—genetics and reproduction—met only a couple of hours a week, and the students considered these snap classes. Three hours a week would also be spent on the behavioral sciences, but these students were so heavily oriented toward physical medicine and disease that they would tend to give this course a low priority also.

Medical students are professional students who know how to study and get passing grades. They are terribly efficient and pragmatic about the way they pursue their studies.

With almost a sixth sense, they immediately identify the difficult courses, determine precisely how much time is justified in mastering each one of them, and then go about parceling out the hours. The behavioral sciences were just not as demanding of time as the hard sciences with their long lists of technical words and formulas to memorize. So the students would downplay them.

Not only did the second semester require less time at school, but the students came back from vacation with a considerable psychological advantage. They had proved to themselves that they could master the required material, no matter how terrifying the demands might appear. They now knew that Penn wasn't trying to flunk them or weed out the best students, the way pre-medical school did.

So freed, the students were now able to turn some of their attention to other areas and consider building a social life.

Last semester, study had got top priority in Matt Lotysh's life, just as it had among most of the students in his class. Now he wanted to fix up his house and go out with some nurses with whom he'd become friendly.

Randy Wiest came back from a vacation of camping with classmates in Canada. Now he intended to spend a lot of time with a classmate he had gotten to know on the trip—Marge Sharmonsky.

Rikki Lights would do a lot more writing, but it would be a difficult year for her as Ron's kidneys continued to deteriorate.

The atmosphere in the classrooms and hallways was decidedly more friendly during the start of the second semester than at any time before. Friendships made during the weeks of final exams—with the pressures and anxieties of studying bringing people together—were apparently flourishing.

Cliques formed along the lines of sporting interests, sex, and race had emerged, though the boundaries weren't firmly drawn. Several of the small groups of companions were former partners from the dissection tables. Things looked so good on this January of 1975. It was almost as though the students had gone home, discovered that the real world was still there, that it was nice, and they didn't want to foresake it all for medicine —at least not just yet.

During the coming months the class would be brought together in a common cause—fighting plans by the school to increase tuition by more than 25 percent. They would, of course, lose the fight but find a uniting purpose for a moment.

The students would also make the sad discovery that they were not so united on a much more basic front—sex. Many of the men would find the women excessively cool and aggressive. And many of the women would find the men immature and naïve.

9

The class of '78 had 48 women, more women than any other class in the school's history. All of them were intelligent and well educated, many were very pretty and only eight were married. With 110 comparatively attractive young men, the prospects for much dating and relating between the sexes appeared great. But there wasn't much at all.

Now that they had more time for socializing during the second semester, the students became increasingly aware of this lack as the weeks passed and the frustration built up.

□ □ □

The male students were seated around a large table in the rooftop restaurant of the Hilton Hotel, griping about the sad state of affairs between the sexes. Stretched out below them in the darkening dusk was the Penn campus and the HUP, directly across from the new hotel.

"The women in the class don't want to be equal to the men," one of them said. "They want to be superior." All of the five men at the table nodded in agreement with pained expressions on their faces as though it were such a waste.

"Yeah, that's it exactly," said a black student who until this moment had been quiet. "The first impression you get from the women is that they don't like being women and they don't like you being a man."

"These women have a high degree of inhibition," a twenty-four-year-old classmate sitting next to him interjected. "They're serious all the time."

Again the heads nodded as he told about one tedious date with a woman classmate who would talk only about medical school matters. He remembered with dread the lengthy pauses in the conversation that made the hours drag.

"Yeah," said the first student. "I don't think many of them like us."

The waiter came and took the students' orders. The dinner was a special occasion for the students, accustomed to eating in cheaper school cafeterias, but none of them ordered anything to drink because it was a week night and they'd all be studying after dinner.

The conversation finally drifted off the main topic of female classmates when one of the men started talking about how he had taken to haunting the bars on campus where he found women undergrads, who seemed to like medical students.

Still, he confessed, most of the nights produced little in the way of companionship and a lot of hours were spent with other guys shooting the pinball machines.

A few days earlier several women students had come to the same restaurant for a special dinner also, but they talked about the men. The comments were equally uncomplimentary.

"A lot of the men in the class are boring," said one woman to another. "The men are more willing to build their lives around medicine and they talk about nothing else. They're very career motivated."

A woman sitting next to her nodded in almost excited agreement. "All their life they have thought about becoming doctors and nothing else. They don't know what to do when they go out. Like this guy I dated. We went out several times and it became obvious that we were going to be only casual friends. That didn't bother me, but I was curious. So I said to him that at one time I had considered what it would be like going to bed with him and I asked him if he had ever had similar thoughts about me. You know what he said?" the woman asked.

Everyone shook their heads.

"He told me that he was waiting for me to make the first move. Can you believe that?"

Now everyone laughed.

"You know what I think it is?" said another woman in her late twenties, slightly older than the others at the table. "The men are self-conscious about sex and about talking about it. Anything to do with sex bothers them. Listen to this one."

Everyone was watching her closely as she told her story.

"I was in the Macke with two guys and we were talking about the lecture on abortion. So I told them that I had had one. They were shocked. You should have seen the expression on their faces. They weren't shocked so much by the fact that I had gotten an abortion but that I should talk about it openly."

All but one of the women smiled knowingly at their companion. The one who didn't smile now spoke.

"The superficiality of the relationships is what bothers me," she said firmly. "I thought about it all through Christmas vacation because I couldn't understand what was wrong. Then I realized it was the superficiality. I talked about it to one guy when I got back and now I'm sorry I did."

She was asked why she was sorry.

"I thought he would agree with me, but instead he said he only had so much time to give. He said he wanted to be friendly, but a woman might want to spend two hours a week relating on a deep level when he might have only one hour to spare. He said he wanted a nondemanding relationship so I said to him, 'What's that?' All meaningful relationships are demanding, but these men don't want demanding relationships."

Women in the class did admit changes in their behavior that could conceivably partly account for the male students' reserved attitudes toward them. But it was far from the whole explanation.

Babies were one matter. Though most of the women intended to raise children as well as practice medicine, they all said that for the moment medicine had top priority.

This bothered one male student who very much wanted children but found his female classmates indifferent to discussing such matters—even as a general topic of conversation, let alone specifically as it would involve them.

One twenty-six-year-old woman student changed in a way that probably would scare off insecure men who needed continual ego stroking.

"Before medical school," she said, "I would do traditional feminine things like being very attentive to the man I was with. He might really be boring or dumb, but I would pretend that he was the smartest and most interesting person I had ever met. I'd pretend to be less bright than I was so he would feel superior and comfortable with me. Now I feel all that stuff is humiliating. I have too much respect for myself now to do things like that just to get a man."

Another student said she changed her style of dress, wearing less-revealing and provocative clothes because she felt they were not appropriate for a medical setting.

Some men said that the women didn't try to look like women but wore only unisex clothes like formless sweaters and slacks. Other male students, however, said that their female classmates used clothing as an aid to be recognized.

One man proposed a rather involved theory, saying: "The women are reverting back to the way they controlled men in their undergraduate days. They wear a dress on these occasions to give them social leverage in an insecure situation, like seeing patients. I feel pity for them because I don't think that it gives them the control that they expect."

Responding to these criticisms, the women said that they dress up for the hospital, just as the men do by wearing ties, because it's expected of them. And they dress sexually conservatively in school because it reflects the seriousness with which they take their careers.

Said one woman student who had formerly been a nurse: "None of us have so strongly developed our professional image that we feel we can carry it off without the help of dressing the role."

□ □ □

Altered behavior patterns by women in a mostly male world may have played a role in the separation between the sexes, but a more important factor was probably the intense pressure the students were under, working ten or more hours a day. Socializing, regardless of sex, had low priority for these students.

A gregarious, twenty-four-year-old Penn graduate gave a party for the entire class early in the year and only forty students came. A little while later he gave another party in his sprawling west Philadelphia home. He announced the party in front of the assembled class, wrote reminders on the blackboard, and personally told everyone he met in the hallway. This time only thirty people showed up, with five men for every woman. One of the two kegs of beer wasn't even tapped.

He thought there was a lot of isolation in the class, but he saw it as a reflection of modern society.

"I just feel that men my age are a lonely bunch," he said. "I feel that a lot of women this age are lonely, too. Everyone thinks that young people are liberated and sexually free, but that isn't so. Many aren't together, are limited sexually. When medical students were undergrads they were the ones who were home studying."

The socializing among the students would improve slightly as they got to know each other better in the second, third, and fourth years.

Oddly the very compactness of the class was inhibiting socializing because medical students tend to be very disapproving of each other's behavior.

If a student openly worked hard to get honors, his classmates would brand him as the typical, excessively compulsive medical school student even though they might be doing the same thing themselves.

The students would be kidded by their peers if they agonized over causing a patient pain when getting blood or if they brooded about the insensitivity of some physicians.

One student was jibbed for the entire first semester because he admitted openly that cadavers and autopsies depressed him and he didn't like dealing with death. Depression was a far less acceptable way of dealing with such fears than making jokes about the cadavers.

Rumors spread through the class with amazing speed and the morning's transgression invariably became the afternoon's rumor.

Time and again students of both sexes cited the confining aspects of the class as an important reason for not getting involved with a class member. Some were worried about the pain of being forced to see the other person day after day in class if the affair were to break up.

One man spoke of how embarrassing it would be to go out with a woman in the class and be judged inadequate, an evaluation he was sure would be prime gossip the day after the date.

"What if you couldn't perform," he said, "if you were impotent with the woman?"

Medical students don't make it through the grind of undergraduate school and pre-med by being rebellious or unmindful of the sensibilities of their peers or superiors.

And the students were as quick to judge as they knew they would be judged.

A lot of the judgments were handed down at the tables in the Macke room, where the students were either talking about medicine or about someone who was not at the table.

The students hoped that their social life would improve in the second year when they reached the hospitals, and the class was no longer a controlling, cohesive entity.

The social life would improve, but mainly because the students would then have a chance to interact with interns, residents, and other students not in their class.

10

For weeks the students had been doing limited physical examinations on each other for practice, but now the time had come for them to examine their first real patient.

Four students were standing in the hallway on one of the internal medicine floors at the HUP, talking to Dr. Joel Morganroth, who would oversee the historic moment. They were wearing their white coats. A penlight and small eye chart stuck out of each breast pocket. And a stethoscope protruded from each right side pocket.

Finally Lois Garner, a small woman with big eyes and an energetic way, asked the question that had been bothering her since they arrived.

"Is it all right," she said in a quiet voice, "to talk in front of the patient about . . . I mean do they know what's wrong with them?" Lois was clutching a new red textbook on physical exams.

Dr. Morganroth nodded. The patients the students would be examining were veteran patients and had been examined many times before for longstanding medical problems, Dr. Morganroth assured Lois.

The four students would be divided into two teams, with one student doing the physical exam and the other getting the medical history.

The students asked some more questions on scholarly topics, but Dr. Morganroth sensed the underlying anxiety that wasn't being expressed in words.

"Don't worry, you'll make a hundred thousand mistakes, but that's what you're here for, to learn. Don't be concerned about inconveniencing or harming the patient, because you won't. You can do everything wrong and you won't cause anyone any difficulty."

Dr. Morganroth was a gentle man, young enough to remember what the students were going through. He smiled and added:

"You're not going to do anything to the patients they haven't agreed to already. That's one of the advantages of going to a teaching hospital, seeing lots of doctors. You might point out something to the doctor on the case that could be useful."

It was a nice thing to say, but these students, who a few weeks earlier couldn't even get a proper blood pressure reading, weren't about to believe they could do anything useful for anyone.

The patient, Mrs. Alabaster, was lying in bed in a pink and white bathrobe when Lois and her teammate, Deborah Spitz, pushed past the curtain separating her from the other patient in the room.

Both students were tense, but the chatty, friendly nature of the white-haired woman put them at rest. Deborah asked the questions for the medical history while Lois began the physical exam.

A thousand thoughts ran through Lois's mind at this moment. Her physical movements must be sure or the patient would detect her anxiety. She had to remember the long list of things to check, moving from head to toe. And she could only hope that if there was an abnormality in, say, the heartbeat or the size of an internal organ that she would be able to recognize it as deviating from the norm.

Deborah continued probing with the questions for the history, but Lois was so preoccupied she didn't hear a word. For many long minutes she held the woman's gnarled hand—joints badly swollen by arthritis—feeling the wrist pulse with the tips of her fingers. It was very irregular and it took Lois almost five minutes to make sure she had recorded it right, much too long with only an hour for a full exam.

Then she wrapped a blood-pressure cuff around Mrs. Alabaster's thin arm, pumped up the device, and listened for the blood to rush through the vessels as she watched the reading on the dial. It read 180.

That seemed too high. Maybe the blood-pressure cuff was put on wrong. So she did it again. This time it read 232.

Lois looked up at Mrs. Alabaster. Fortunately the old woman was too preoccupied answering Deborah's questions to pay attention to Lois. Lois tried a third time to get a reading. It was 232 again. This was hard to believe. Lois didn't know beforehand that the woman had high blood pressure and her readings were right.

A nurse came into the room, looked at the two medical students without smiling or saying a word, and then left as abruptly as she had arrived.

Lois got a blood-pressure reading from the other arm and then repeated the time-consuming process with Mrs. Alabaster sitting up. Already fifteen minutes had passed and she still had a long way to go to complete the exam.

"When did you get the chest pain?" Deborah asked, pushing on with her history-taking. Cheerfully Mrs. Alabaster continued answering the questions as Lois moved on to check her head.

An unidentified doctor pushed past the curtain, reached across the bed for Mrs. Alabaster's arm to check a skin test, and left as abruptly as the nurse had before him. Lois hardly even noticed him.

"You have more doctors than you know what to do with," Deborah said brightly.

"It's a regular parade," Mrs. Alabaster said without turning her head to Deborah because Lois was checking out her eyes. "But that's the way it is when you go to a hospital with a medical school. It's really very good because you get so much attention. Maybe you'll find something the other doctors didn't."

Deborah didn't smile.

Telling Mrs. Alabaster to look straight at her, Lois held her fingers wide apart. Loosening up a bit, Deborah explained that Lois was checking her peripheral vision.

"I know," Mrs. Alabaster said, smiling broadly with the amusement of an older woman who enjoys being doted over. "The doctors who were in here just before you did exactly the same thing."

"Great!" Lois said, warming up now that the exam was progressing faster and Mrs. Alabaster was turning out to be such a charming woman. But Lois still had a lot to do with only thirty minutes left.

Lois couldn't have asked for a better first patient as far as personality was involved, but the irregular pulse and unusually high blood pressure would have unnerved any beginning medical student.

Lois looked at her watch. The time was really rushing by. She still had to check out the chest and heart and all the other internal organs and glands and other things that might reveal disease.

But luck was not with Lois this day, unless it was bad luck.

Lois had just placed her stethoscope on Mrs. Alabaster's chest when the nurse came in with the wheelchair.

It was time to take Mrs. Alabaster down for her x-rays.

Lois couldn't believe it. Deborah couldn't believe it. But it was happening.

The two students tried to convince the nurse to wait. But she wasn't about to let students interfere with the operations of the HUP.

"Oh, I'm so sorry you couldn't finish," Mrs. Alabaster said climbing into the wheelchair. "Maybe you could come back another time, if you wish."

11

The depressing rumor spread through the class so fast that by lunchtime everyone had gotten the word: Tuition was going up by more than 25 percent—from $3,580 a year to $4,500. This was a record increase and the students could hardly believe it.

They discussed it huddled in groups in the hallways and over bad coffee in paper cups in the lunchroom. One student raised the possibility of a strike. Another said that was out of the question.

The outrage and prevailing sense of impotence were expressed openly at a meeting with Dean Stemmler that evening in the medical students' lounge.

About a hundred students sat in chairs and sofas and on the floor of the carpeted lounge as the dean led them through the wonderland of university financing with the aid of tables flashed on a movie screen.

They listened quietly for about a half hour and then the questions came.

Why couldn't the medical school cut faculty salaries rather than raising tuition?

Wouldn't it be cheaper to sever ties with the university and go it alone? Maybe the school should discontinue or reduce partial scholarships given to the children of university professionals as a fringe benefit.

Could the physicians at the HUP get their more affluent patients to contribute to a loan fund to help medical students?

One by one, the suggestions were disposed of by the dean as being impractical or improper or impossible. And then he got to his main point, the basic truth that explained why tuition was going up so much and why things were going to get worse and why the students should not expect much help from the outside:

"There is no sympathy for medical students. The mood of the country is not to support medical education."

He made the statement with a calmness that only heightened its impact. This was not a matter that could be debated.

Congress is thinking of reducing its aid to medical education, he continued, and the state aid of $4,400 per student was not secure.

After more than two hours, the meeting ended as most academic meetings end: A faculty-student committee was established. But no one really expected it to resolve major issues.

Many students left the lounge that night with a depressing and angry sense of isolation, cut off from the university, faculty, and the rest of the world that did not seem to care about their problems.

"If they [society] screw me," one student said to the dean after the meeting broke up, "then when the time comes I'm going to get mine."

This sense of vengeance was held by only a few students, but it was more prevalent than it was seven months earlier, when the students started classes.

It was becoming not at all uncommon to hear students cite the long hours and high cost of training as an explanation—if not justification—for the high fees that doctors charged.

Idealism is put to the test—and sometimes to rest—in medical school. At this embryonic stage in his professional life, the medical student must endure the loneliness and the burden of work it takes to become a physician without the prestige or financial rewards of the profession.

With only one seat for every three applicants, a student has to work hard to get into medical school. And once there, he has to work much harder than other graduate students to get a degree, accumulating on the average a $20,000 debt along the way.

For four years he must live at subsistence level. Then he faces three or four more years of hospital training, where he can earn no more than $12,000 to $16,000 a year. As an intern, he will work eighty hours a week or more, only a little less as a resident.

At the age of thirty, almost a decade after most other people have started earning a living, the doctor is ready to open his own practice and start making money.

The typical specialist, and most doctors these days are specialists, has gone through four years of undergradaute school, four years of medical school, and three or four years of residency training. It's an investment of eleven years of education and training after leaving high school.

Becoming a physician is rough, but sympathy is tempered by the realization that most medical students come from comfortable backgrounds and that all of them are entering the most lucrative of all professions, with the average doctor making $55,000 a year.

Until recently the future and expectations of the prospective physician were secure. But today's student begins his career at a historic and, for her or him, disquieting moment. For the first time, the profession's traditional autonomy is being challenged, and large segments of the field are coming under the control of nonphysicians.

The students fear, and for good cause, that by the time they finish school the government will control their futures either indirectly—through national health insurance, which is on the verge of being passed—or through outright restrictions on the types of doctors that may be trained.

Unlike those who went before them, today's students may not be able to choose a specialty. They may have to be content with becoming the type of doctor that society says it needs.

Threatening to control the physician's career at one end, society is also considering pulling back financial support at the other end. The growing feeling is that medical students should pay for a larger percentage of what it costs to educate them, since they will eventually enjoy the rewards of a lucrative profession.

It costs twice as much to train a doctor as it does to produce other professionals, such as lawyers and architects, and three to four times as much as educating an undergradaute student.

The $3,580 that the Penn student paid for tuition was only a fifth of what it actually cost to provide that education. The costs are high because medical education requires many laboratory courses, clinical instruction, and a faculty ratio of almost one to one.

Because of the large subsidization, medical students used to pay about the same for tuition as all other graduate students. But now the university was increasing the tuition of medical students more than 25 percent, compared with an average boost of about 10 percent for other graduate students.

It was a nationwide trend, and just beginning. Before the class of '78 graduated, the tuition at Penn would reach $6,000. In 1978 the national average for private medical school tuitions was $5,334, and at Georgetown University, in the District of Columbia, the highest tuition of all would be paid—$12,500 a year.

Even at the old tuition rate of $3,590, medical school was an expensive business. It involved a bewildering array of loan programs some of which were available only to minority students or persons willing to serve as military physicians or public officers for four years.

Penn's tour guide through this labyrinth of indebtedness was Robert d'Augustine, assistant director of graduate financial aid, who dispensed the institutional largess with disturbing equanimity.

It had been determined that a single student needed only $7,100 for the ten months he spent at Penn in 1975. The typical student put together the $7,100 with $3,500 in various scholarships, $2,900 in government and private loans, and $700 saved from summer employment.

In computing loans and scholarships, the university allowed a married student a budget of $8,650 a year plus $600 for children. If the student's spouse made money, that income was deducted from some of the scholarships and loans that the student was eligible for.

This might seem to be a generous allotment, but more than half of the single student's budget went for the $3,580 tuition, and a couple of hundred dollars went for books, instruments, and other supplies. This did not leave much for entertainment or other luxuries.

Some students beat these high costs with a military scholarship that paid for tuition and provided $400 a month in living expenses. The catch was that the students would have to give the military one year of service for every year of subsidy.

Even with this requirement, the scholarships were so much in demand that no more were available even though the military services had a total of five thousand to offer. In past years they went begging.

Two students were getting full scholarships as part of a federal program designed to encourage science-research-oriented physicians. They would graduate with Ph.Ds as well as M.Ds, but they would have to go to school for six years.

Most students would go through medical school in four years, but would leave it heavily in debt—$20,000 for the typical student.

Payment of the loan principal usually could be put off until the student finished residency training four or five years after graduation. But then he had to pay $200 a month for the next ten years, d'Augustine said.

Some students go much deeper into debt because they want more than the meager life allowed by the formula student budgets. One older graduate student had lived the financially strained life of a student practically all his adult life and was tired of it. So he borrowed way over the guidelines and would amass a $45,000 debt by 1978.

Matt Lotysh got by with the aid of food stamps, which paid for everything except rent, and set aside $15.00 a week for meals, which included a lot of hamburger and chicken.

"You get just enough money to exist and fulfill your function as a medical student," said Marc Micozzi, twenty-one.

"They don't take into account that you have to maintain your human traits," he said, adding that it's a "psychologically simple thing" to fall into the routine of getting up, going to school, studying, and going to sleep, almost unaware that no money is available for doing anything else.

Students from wealthy families would obviously have an easier time of it, but d'Augustine and Dr. Richard Schwarz, head of the admissions committee, insisted that a student's family background and financial resources had nothing to do with whether he or she was admitted. Admissions officers were instructed to ignore parental occupations in making a judgment, Dr. Schwarz said, and family income was not even known until after the student had been admitted.

The only advantage the son of a physician had was that if his father or mother was a Penn alumnus she or he would be given the edge when competing against an equally qualified applicant. But this close a tie happened rarely, Dr. Schwarz said. He assumed that the reason medical school had so many middle-class students, and so many children of physicians, was that they were motivated to become doctors and had the culturally and genetically endowed intelligence to do it.

Most important, perhaps, they knew that becoming a physician was a possible thing for them to do—not a wild unrealistic dream, a negative perspective that discouraged many minority students and, until recently, even most women.

One black woman student had good reason not to contemplate a medical career. Tuition cost more than her mother made in a year. But the big advantage the student had was a mother who insisted that her daughter could become a physician if she was determined enough.

Like most stereotypes, the stereotype of a medical student in this country has factual components. Chances are that the medical student does have at least a physically comfortable life growing up, and that he will make a lot of money when he starts practicing on his own.

In 1975, the median net income for young, office-based physicians was about $50,000, ranging from $43,060 to $66,750, according to a survey by the professional journal *Medical Economics*. Comparable figures came from the American Medical Association.

But, like most stereotypes, this one ignores subtleties that can profoundly affect public attitudes. Unfortunately, many decisions made in the public arena are based upon stereotypes.

"I don't question that medical school is a good investment," said Steve Levine, a member of the first-year-class student government. "I don't mind paying my own way through medical school," he continued. "I wouldn't even mind paying the full twenty thousand or whatever it costs society to educate us, but I can't pay it now."

This was the heavy concern of most medical students then, especially with announcements of tuition increases. But, Steve pointed out, it was a tremendous stress seeing the indebtedness grow with no money coming in, and no assurance that adequate loan money would continue to be available. It was an economic catch-22, where the student had to go further into debt to get out of debt.

If for some reason—financial, personal, medical—the student did not finish and get a medical degree, he would be left with a huge debt and very limited means to pay it back. This stress, on top of the stairs of hard work and long hours, pinned the student's future to the wall.

But the redeeming factor, and it's a big one, was that if he stuck it out and became a doctor, the future he was pinned to should be a very nice one.

12

Faint fringes of green were beginning to outline the trees on Hamilton Walk and the days were decidedly beginning to feel warmer. Spring was arriving. And it felt good to be young, a medical student, and finally on the way.

The mass of material being absorbed had yet to form an intellectually cohesive whole. The students' knowledge was spotty and the information hadn't started to overlap, so they were yet to feel secure in the extent of their mastery.

But they were beginning to have a sense of the human body and how it worked and how disease stopped it from working properly. The mechanism of the disease process was being revealed to them.

They already knew from physiology how the normal body was supposed to work. Pathology examined the disease process and histology took them into the minute and dynamic world of the trillions of cells that make up the human body.

Now in the second semester they were learning in their biochemistry and neurobiology courses how the body's functions were influenced or controlled by the nerves and chemicals in the body. And the pharmacology courses would show how all of this could be influenced with drugs.

The students were beginning to speak the physician's language and they were learning to think the way physicians think—objectively, in terms of cause and effect.

Repetition had smoothed away the clumsiness so that now the students were putting on blood-pressure cuffs with authority and the thumping of the normally beating heart was being recognized without doubt as the students grew accustomed to having stethoscopes plugged into their ears.

Pain, death, and fear were still enemies to be feared, but the students were beginning to accept them more readily now and soon they would find pain an ally, an important clue in assessing the distress of their patients.

The students didn't have to dread the approach of the final weeks of the term because of finals, as they did during the first semester. They were taking finals at eight-week intervals as the various sections of courses were completed.

It indeed was turning out to be a much more humane semester than the first one.

□ □ □

Ron was beginning to experience terrible pains in his joints and his arms were feeling heavy. He tired easily and kept running out of breath. In Atlantic City, during a jazz concert at which he was performing, Ron had to run to the bathroom to throw up. His disease was getting worse. Soon his kidneys would stop working completely.

Finally his physician, Dr. Robert Grossman, who ran the kidney dialysis unit at the HUP, told Ron that he would have to start thinking about going on the machine. It was a much more fearful thought for Rikki than Ron because she had seen the dialysis unit and had been reading up on the machine.

She knew that the attrition rate was 10 percent per year. That meant that 10 percent of the patients tied to the machine died each year. Theoretically everyone would be dead at the end of ten years. Ron was only twenty-six.

In the coming months, Rikki would become an expert on kidney disease, dialysis, and dealing with the stress of terminal illness. For the moment, she and Ron hoped to put off the day when he would go on the machine as long as possible.

But the relentless disease wasn't giving them much time. Ron was getting weaker and the drugs to control his blood pressure and other problems were making the normally cheerful man depressed. And it was becoming increasingly harder for him to find the strength to sit at his beloved drums.

□ □ □

The second semester would be the best months of the whole four years for Marge Shamonsky and Randy Wiest. They were falling in love. Instead of going to the books every weekend as they had in the first semester, Randy and Marge were frequently with each other on hikes and camping trips.

Now they were looking forward to the approaching trout season. The first year of school would be almost over then, a delicious thought to contemplate as they waited for the fish to bite.

Unfortunately the second year in the hospitals would be very disappointing for Marge, who would find the impersonal and anonymous nature of the teaching institution more than she could take. Eventually she would confront her doubts and decide to leave medical school. But Marge had no hint of this trouble as spring approached during this first year in school when everything was looking so beautiful to her.

□ □ □

Ron Cargill was not doing so well. His fiancée was beginning to balk at the long hours he spent both in school and on the ghetto street corners of

Camden and Philadelphia, where he preached the word of the Black Muslims, who were helping him through school. Soon the engagement would be broken off.

He was spending virtually all his time either studying or proselytizing. Going from the slums to the elite University of Pennsylvania School of Medicine strictly on his own ability, Ron was an excellent role model to tempt the disillusioned, aimless youth of the ghetto streets.

Ron had succeeded in isolating himself from more than just the rest of the class. In his Chicago gangster, broad-brimmed hat, he looked so different from everyone else that it was causing problems for him. Several times the police had stopped and frisked him, thinking he was the rapist they were looking for, or a suspicious character about to do no good. Rarely would Ron leave his apartment without his university ID. Once the university security patrol even grabbed him and threw him up against the wall in front of his classmates when the guards saw him coming in a back door late at night. The usual entrance had been locked and the broad-brimmed hat coming through the other door prompted a Pavlovian response on the part of the police.

Matt Lotysh was also unhappy. The grind was getting to him and he tired of all the lectures. He longed for the operating room and heart surgery, which was the goal that had brought him to medical school in the first place.

He also longed for California and the warm weather and the swimming deep down into the ocean for the abalone. The only thing that was keeping up his spirits was the popularity of medical students among women.

Wherever he went, the gregarious Matt Lotysh seemed to be running into women who wanted to go out with him. He wasn't bad-looking, he was very personable, and appeared sincere and interested in the people he spoke to, and above all he was a young man with a very attractive future.

"It's amazing what it's like," he said, describing it to a friend. "You meet women everywhere. Anywhere. You just name it. Unbelievable. You meet one nurse and she has two friends. One of them likes to screw. She has two friends. Both of them like to screw. One of them invites you to a party. Three girls there. One leaves early and gives you her phone number. One goes off with somebody else. You remember her name. You see her again and get a date. The third you go home with. It's like a family tree."

It sounded like a bachelor's utopia, but Matt could only count the days until the first year was over. He wanted to get to the hospitals.

In only a few weeks the first year would be over and everyone would be going to the hospitals.

13

The final hours of their first year ticked away as the students began arriving. It was 8:30 A.M., Friday, June 13—hopefully not an unlucky sign for the pharmacology examination that would begin in thirty minutes.

Even though the test, the last one of the year, would not begin for a while, many students were already sitting in the laboratory rooms where the written tests would be given, going over their notes for the last time.

Barbara Turner, who would spend her summer working at the famed Peter Bent Brigham Hospital in Boston, arrived on a bicycle, locked it to the fence in front of the medical school and went in for the test.

Victor E. Battles was feeling pretty good. He had done fairly well on the midterm examinations and was confident. Carrying no books, Colin Kerr looked carefree as he strode down the hall on his long legs.

With the exception of a three-week vacation at Christmas time, the students had been going to school almost constantly, thirty-one hours or more a week, since September 3. Studying twenty to thirty more hours a week, they had found it a heavy grind; but the first year was almost over now.

In some ways, it was a sad day because it would be the last time that they would work together as a class. Next year they would be individually assigned to different hospitals, and they would not come together again as a unit until 1978 on graduation day.

Given in four different lab rooms, the pharmacology tests started roughly in unison, as some students trailed in late. Pharmacology is difficult but a very important course. The students were given 212 true-or-false questions.

Because they had been taking tests all term long, instead of just during the final week, this last week was not particularly difficult. Pharmacology was the only exam anyone was very worried about.

□ □ □

The *esprit de corps* of the class had been a variable thing during the first year. They had come together almost ten months ago as strangers, and now they were finishing up fairly well acquainted with one another.

Some had arrived hopeful and left alienated after the first year. Others felt good about the class the moment they started in September and felt even better about it now. Most of them felt good at times and negative at others.

The class had come together as a social unit only a few weeks earlier for a revue, "Freshman Follies," a musical variety show followed by a beer and wine party in the student lounge that lasted past 3:00 A.M.

It was almost as though the students were just looking for an excuse to get together for something other than medicine. More than one-third of the class had taken part in writing and acting in the production, which parodied everything—from undergraduate women who study in the medical library in the hope of finding a medical student husband to professors who cannot stay awake during their own lectures.

They danced almost continuously all night, and for one brief whirl they were having fun with one another to the exclusion of everything else.

Downstairs in a hallway, away from the noise of the party, a student sat on the ground between two gray steel lockers, playing back the tapes of the revue they had just enacted.

"It's a shame that it's ending now," he said, looking sad, "just when the class all came together."

Two students who were particularly positive in their attitudes about the class were Randy Wiest and Marge Shamonsky. They had told everyone that they were going to get married in August. It had taken only a few months of camping and studying together for Randy and Marge to realize that they were special to each other. Eagerly they would look forward to the weekends when they could escape from the city and its confining atmosphere and enjoy the outdoors together.

At those times Penn and medical school and the stiff, formal structure of the hospitals seemed so many miles away and they felt so comfortable enjoying the same things. Marriage was inevitable even though it was scary. Randy had proposed to Marge on the first day of the trout season.

□ □ □

The test was not difficult.

Colin Kerr was one of the first to finish, leaving in less than ninety minutes.

With a big smile on his face, Matt Lotysh emerged from one of the test rooms, took a drink of water, and returned to finish up. The answers to the questions were coming to him without effort.

Rikki Lights was happy but preoccupied. Ron was in the hospital again. Rikki had planned to read some of her poetry at the International Women's Year conference in Mexico City, but now she had decided to stay in Philadelphia with Ron.

The party atmosphere with champagne and laughter that had ended the first semester did not mark the end of the second term. Some of the students gathered in the Macke, but most of them spoke to one another only briefly in the hallway and left.

Helene Silverblatt checked her mailbox—the grades from other classes were awaiting her—and talked to some classmates before going home. She would fly to Peru Wednesday, where she would help her anthropologist-sister do field work.

Many students would spend the summer working in hospitals or other medical facilities, where they would make some money and view the practice of medicine from a different perspective. Others would spend the summer in school, getting a vacation of only a few weeks.

Walter Tsou, for one, would spend eight weeks of July and August doing his surgical clerkship. In September, he and many of the other students would take the first part of the national boards—exams that would be given to students throughout the country.

By 1:00 P.M., most of the students had left the campus. A few parties would be given later in the day. The black students would have a lunch party on the top floor of the nearby Hilton Hotel. But most of the students would just go on their way.

It was getting warmer outside. Hamilton Walk was beautiful. The first year was over.

14

Ron's condition continued to deteriorate throughout the summer. It was becoming increasingly difficult for him and Rikki to deny that one day he would have to go on the machine.

Ron could hardly move about without becoming immediately exhausted. He was vomiting every day now. Rikki knew what these symptoms meant. But she kept trying to deny them to herself. Maybe it was a chronic stomach upset or indigestion, she said to herself, anything but uremia. But it was uremia.

His kidneys were unable to clear toxic wastes from his blood and the poisons were building up to the point where his body couldn't tolerate them. He was on a strict diet now to hold down the amount of work his ailing kidneys had to do. But now his kidneys weren't even up to meeting this reduced demand.

Finally, in July, Dr. Grossman told Ron and Rikki that the time had come to put in the fistula. It was not a difficult procedure. The surgeons merely cut into the skin of Ron's left arm and sewed the artery to the vein in such a way that they could be hooked up to the kidney machine.

Though the surgical procedure was small, the psychological impact was massive. Every time Ron looked at the healing wound in his left arm he was reminded of the fact that he was no longer a complete human being, a self-sufficient organism capable of surviving without dependence on outside things like the kidney machine.

Even so, all through the summer Ron clung to the thought that he would never have to go on the machine, that the fistula was just a precaution. But the relentless progress of the disease continued, and finally, in the autumn, Dr. Grossman told him that the time had come. He would have to go on the machine now. Denial was no longer possible.

Years later Rikki would still remember the impact of discovering that her dear friend would have to start dialysis and be dependent upon a machine for the rest of his life.

"It was like an earthquake," she said, "with this ragged crack spreading across the ground. You have only seconds to jump and if you're too slow, you end up falling in the crack . . . lost."

Both Ron and Rikki had to incorporate the thought of being kept alive
by a machine into their thinking, into their images of self. Life was no longer
a boundless future; it was circumscribed by both time and geography.

The machine to which Ron would find himself linked looked something
like a washing machine—and in a sense it was one. Large-bore needles—
almost an eighth of an inch in diameter—would be stuck into the artery
and vein. Blood from the artery would go through the needle into the tube
through which it would be taken to the dialysis unit, cleansed of impurities,
and passed into Ron's body through the needle implanted in his vein.

This would happen from 7:00 A.M. to 2:00 P.M. every Tuesday, Thursday, and Saturday. Ron could not be away from the machine for more than
two days or the toxins in his blood would reach a dangerous level.

But there was one hope—kidney transplantation. Rikki knew the statistics well. She was fast becoming the best-informed kidney specialist in
her class. There were good statistics and there were bad statistics.

Only 42 percent of the kidneys transplanted from persons who had
died—so-called cadaver transplants—were still functioning two years after
implantation. Fifty-eight percent of the organs were rejected by the recipient's natural immunity, which attacks the foreign kidney just as it
would threatening bacteria or viruses. But the survival rate for kidneys
donated by a genetically similar relative was almost double that—73 percent.

Ron's thirty-one-year-old brother, James, a conga player in the band,
had offered one of his kidneys. The doctors at the HUP would run tests to
see if Jim and Ron's tissue were compatible. Just as brothers may have different blood types, making transfusions between them impossible, so they
may have different tissue types. If the tissues matched well, then a transplant
would be feasible.

Rikki was delighted to know that at least this possibility existed. But
she also knew that transplantation was not without problems. Again her
growing knowledge repressed her optimism.

She knew that transplant patients had to take drugs that would depress
their natural immunity. This was designed to prevent their bodies from re-
jecting the donated kidney. But the drugs also unfortunately made the patients susceptible to other diseases like colds, pneumonia, a variety of infections, and cancer.

Every hope seemed tarnished with a disappointment. It had been like
this for more than a year—ever since Dr. Chirico made the sad diagnosis.
For months now, Rikki and Ron had been talking about marriage, but each
time they got ready to go ahead with it another medical calamity would
strike.

Enough was enough. They would get married now in February regardless of what happened.

15

The second year of medical school would be sharply different from anything the students had done so far in their seventeen- to twenty-year-long educational careers.

With the exception of their once-a-week afternoon visits to the hospitals, the first year of medical school was just like undergraduate school, the days filled with lectures, laboratory work, and seminars.

Now the students were going to the hospitals for clinical training. Most medical schools in the United States keep the students in the classrooms for the first two years before providing clinical training, but Penn revised its curriculum in 1968, abbreviating required lecture courses in the basic sciences, increasing the number of electives, and getting students into the hospitals quicker so that they could appreciate the value of the information they were laboring to master.

Now in the second year the students would begin to do the things that physicians did in the real world. They would now see all the abstract knowledge in a very real sense, applied to patients with feelings, personalities, and human needs just like their own.

Surprisingly, the bulk of medical schooling still consists of that one old educational standby, apprenticeship training—learning at the elbow of someone doing the thing the novice must learn.

The students would be individually assigned to the seven hospitals affiliated with Penn's teaching program. Most of the clerkships, as this training is called, would involve one-month rotations through various specialty services at the different hospitals. The two broadest clerkships—in surgery and medicine—would last eight weeks.

The students still had to take the equivalent of four months of classwork in basic sciences. But from now on the bulk of their work would involve clerkships, the number being variable, depending on the student's interest.

To graduate, they had to amass thirty-two points—with one point equal to one month of study or an average rotation. Most of the students would rotate through fifteen to twenty services. Students who wanted to work eleven-month years could fulfill their requirements in three years and graduate a year early—nine of the students in the class of '78 would do just that. Others could work at a more leisurely pace and spend five years in school. It didn't matter to Penn. Whether the students stayed in school for three, four, or five years they would pay four years' worth of tuition.

Medical education is not a sequential learning experience. That is, the students don't learn progressively more complex things, going from the first year to the fourth, though they are trusted to do more difficult things as they gain experience.

The second, third, and fourth years of medical school don't even exist as identifiable entities. A year doesn't start in September and end in June. The three years blend into a single continuum that finally ends with graduation. A student might just as likely be doing a clerkship in the middle of the August vacation period as in December or January.

It's difficult to tell from the courses being taken what year a student happens to be in. Medical education is more or less a smorgasbord of learning, with the students sampling different dishes in no particular order as they wander through the hospitals.

One student might take Pediatrics 200 in the second year and OB-GYN 200 in the third year and another might do the reverse.

Some advanced clerkships, the "300" courses, do require prior experience. For instance, a student couldn't take Medicine 300, which is almost like being a junior intern, without first taking Medicine 200, the introductory clerkship to internal medicine. But the difference between the "200" and "300" courses is not so much what the student learns as it is how much responsibility the student is given.

In any case, the amount of freedom students have in caring for patients is small. They can't prescribe medicine. They can't institute therapy of any sort without the concurrence of the intern or resident above them. Practically the only invasive procedures they are allowed to do is draw blood, a thing they do a lot, do rectal and pelvic examinations, give shots (ordered by someone else), and perhaps do a few minor sutures.

Students will take medical histories from patients, but the intern will repeat them. The student's physical exam is repeated by someone else. In fact, the student's absence or presence does not materially affect the care of the patient, though they do do a lot of mundane work that other people don't want to do.

Medical education is a highly organized tier system of expertise being passed down from one level to the next. At the bottom of the pyramid are the "200" students who learn from the "300" students, interns, residents, nurses, and frequently even the patients. The intern, or first-year resident, is the lowest-ranking physician, only one year ahead of the fourth-year student. He doesn't have a license to practice medicine yet, but he has a medical degree and hence is entitled to be called doctor.

(Students are frequently called doctors by patients and it's rarely corrected. In fact, the mistake is encouraged, with physicians introducing students as "student doctors." They might even go so far as to call a student "Dr. Jones" in front of the patients.)

The intern has the right to prescribe medicine and institute therapy on his own. He has the legal authority and obligation to care for the patient, and in a teaching institution much of his time is spent showing students what to do.

Above the intern is the second-year resident, who is a licensed physician but practices medicine only in the hospital. He takes care of patients directly, but he also oversees the care provided by the interns under him.

Finally there is the attending physician. These are full-fledged physicians, including full professors, who have private patients, hold high-level teaching positions, and perhaps even have national reputations.

The attendings see patients, but usually only during rounds once a day, unless their personal patients happen to be on the service they are covering in their roles as teachers. Usually the attendings are consulted only on the more difficult day-to-day problems the residents encounter.

And who is above the attending? Actually no one as far as the day-to-day care of the patient is concerned. But in teaching institutions there are people intellectually above the attendings in highly specialized areas. These are the specialists' specialists, the superstars, the research heroes, who each week conduct a thing called grand rounds, at which everyone, from the students on up to the attendings, hears the latest word on some disease or problem.

Sometimes grand rounds are conducted by people in the hospital or school. It's something of an honor to present grand rounds. At other times the expert may be a nationally renowned figure who might have traveled halfway around the world to help expand the growing mountain of knowledge that is hopefully slowly advancing medical care.

16

Mark Reber sat amid the busy activity of the nurses' station, hunched over Nelson's *Textbook of Pediatrics*. He was hurriedly reviewing the section on rheumatic disease.

A six-year-old girl was being admitted to Children's Hospital with possible chorea and she would be Mark's patient—and he wanted to be ready when the girl and her parents arrived in a few minutes.

Chorea is not a disease, but a symptom—a muscular twitching. In a child this age, it is usually caused by rheumatic fever, but it is important to be sure. It would be tragic to condemn a child unnecessarily to twenty years of antibiotic therapy and the fear of heart disease when in fact she was not suffering from rheumatic disease.

Mark finished the chapter, went over the section describing chorea one more time, and closed the big green textbook. It had been more than a half hour since the admitting office called, and the girl still had not arrived. Mark got up and went looking for the intern he was working under.

□ □ □

With the first year of study behind them now, the students seemed a lot more comfortable with their roles as members of the medical team, and now they frequently were being mistaken for full-fledged doctors as they moved about the hospitals in their short white coats.

Since they were contributing to patient care in a small way this year, they no longer thought of themselves as imposing on patients when they questioned them for medical histories or conducted physical exams.

Many students gained practical experience during the summer working in low-paid hospital or research jobs, and a few got a headstart on the rest of the class by taking summer courses.

Walter Tsou, who seemed so young last year with his University of Pennsylvania Streaking Team shirt, had become much quieter and more self-assured. He spent the summer helping in an operating room learning the many things surgery can and cannot do for sick people.

Jim Nestor liked to tell people how he worked during the summer in the maintenance department of Hahnemann Hospital, giving people the impression he swept floors. Actually, he had done professional work as a certified engineer.

Helene Silverblatt did not return to school for the first part of the fall session but stayed on in Peru an extra month, doing field work with her anthropologist-sister. She would start classes later in the fall.

Matt Lotysh was as bouncing and energetic as ever, still filled with the wonder of where he had come from and where he was going. Matt's summer had been spent doing work in genetics at Children's Hospital, "a fantastic, exhausting eight weeks," he said.

Of the 160 students who had come together for the first time in that humid Penn lecture hall the year before, only three had left school—two for psychiatric reasons and one on a temporary leave. Five new students, one a woman, joined the class this year, transferring from other medical schools.

□ □ □

Little six-year-old Susan Loyd did not look sick at all as she bounced up and down in the crib, crying to be taken to the ward playroom, which the women in the admitting office had told her about.

It was hard to believe that this happy child might have a serious disease that was disrupting her neurologic system, causing her to jerk in a strange if not grotesque manner.

Sitting next to the crib, in plastic chairs, Susan's mother, along with Mark Reber, tried to discuss her problem.

"I didn't think much of it in the beginning," Mrs. Loyd said. She referred to Susan's jerking movements, in which the girl drew in her chin against her throat like a horse being reined in sharply. "I thought maybe it was something on TV she was imitating. But then last week she complained of a sore throat. . . ."

Ordinarily the sore throat would have suggested rheumatic fever in such a case, but it came after the movements began, so the connection was unlikely. Mark noted the sequence on the clipboard resting in his lap.

Mrs. Loyd said that Susan's pediatrician prescribed antibiotics and took a throat culture, which subsequently turned out to be negative. Susan had a slight fever, but it did not seem very bad, Mrs. Loyd said. But then the arm movements began.

"Arm movements?" Mark asked.

"She'd jerk out her arms—like that," the mother said, looking up suddenly at Susan.

Susan was standing up in the crib, drawing in her neck and twisting her arm with spastic movements. Mark looked at her, and she did it again for him. Mark made another note on his clipboard and continued with the interview.

Other than getting many colds the year before, when Susan started school, and the fact that the mother was unusually conscientious about medical care, nothing else in the history seemed remarkable to the medical student. Mark stood up, thanked the mother, and played gently with Susan for a moment.

The softness of the moment in the dimly lit room was broken a few seconds later when Mark took them into the harshly lighted treatment room with its bustle of nurses and doctors. Mark examined Susan but he was double-checked by the intern, Dr. Laurence Ashbacher, who drew blood and took samples from Susan's throat and nose for testing.

"Do you think it's serious?" Mrs. Loyd asked after the exam was over and Susan had gone to the playroom.

Dr. Ashbacher conceded that it could be serious, but said that they would have to wait for the lab tests and other studies.

"Is it contagious?" she asked. "Could she choke herself when she does this thing? I mean, like if she did it when she was eating something?" Many other questions were asked, but each time Mark and Dr. Ashbacher had to give incomplete or tentative answers.

"You'll tell us, won't you, as soon as you know?" Mrs. Loyd asked, looking intently into Dr. Ashbacher's eyes. "If it's something serious, you'll let us know?"

Dr. Ashbacher squeezed Mrs. Loyd's arm in response.

"Don't worry," he said. "We'll let you know as soon as we know anything. We won't hold any shots back from you."

□ □ □

Before Susan's admission, Mark's first week on the pediatric rotation at Children's Hospital had been uneventful. Most of the time was spent attending lectures and getting to know the people and hospital routine.

Mark, and classmate Robert Busch, a smiling, eager youth of twenty-two who freely showed his excitement and enthusiasm, had been assigned to one of the two teams covering the "baby ward" on the fifth floor.

It was a hectic place filled with nurses, parents who slept on cots next to their sick children, and herds of specialists and students trooping in and out of the dozen rooms that constitute the ward.

The head of Mark's team was a third-year resident, Dr. Sally Haggerty, a friendly, informal, comfortable woman of twenty-eight. Dr. Haggerty led her team with an inconspicuous authority that was apparent only when she gently corrected one of those under her.

Dr. Ashbacher was almost Dr. Haggerty's opposite. A driven twenty-six-year-old honors graduate, Dr. Ashbacher worked with a relentless self-assurance that left little time for imperfection or the ineptness of insecure medical students.

The four-week rotation through pediatrics was required of all Penn medical students, half of whom would never again see children as patients, except, perhaps, in an emergency room.

After the four weeks, the students would in no way be competent to treat children, but hopefully they would at least be able to examine a well child and realize some of the important differences between caring for a child and caring for an adult.

The sick babies filling the sixty beds and isolettes on the ward represented both the successes and failures of pediatric medicine. Several babies were alive only because of medical progress that had been made in recent years. And some were dying because that progress had not been enough.

The status of this battle between medical science and disease was reviewed each day on morning and evening bed rounds. Leading her small entourage of nurses, doctors, and students, Dr. Haggerty would move from crib to crib, pausing only long enough to look at each baby from a distance and listen to the intern's shorthand description of the baby's condition and planned care. "Baby Girl Schaefer is all ready to go home now, but they can't contact the mother," the intern said to Dr. Haggerty, who smiled at the baby bouncing up and down happily in her crib. The antibiotics had knocked out the baby's meningitis but the social services department was unable to reach the mother, who had been in to see her daughter only once in the preceding week.

Dr. Haggerty sighed and moved on to the next crib. "Ah, Bobby looks fine today," she said brightening. "He's really coming along very nicely. We might get him off the machine yet."

She referred to Baby Boy Taylor, a favorite of the ward because he had been there since his birth eleven months earlier. They were weaning him off the respirator that had been breathing for him all his life. Born with hyaline membrane disease, the same lung condition that killed President Kennedy's baby, his life was saved by a technique developed during the last three years.

"He was such a small little thing when he was born," Dr. Haggerty said, leading on to the next room, where all the baby isolettes were. "You never would have thought that he'd make it. But he's doing very nicely."

Dr. Haggerty peered into an isolette glowing with a bright light inside. Lying under the eerie blue light with her eyes bandaged for protection, two-day-old Baby Girl Marter was responding well to the therapy and her jaundice was disappearing. Shining through her thin skin, the light photochemically broke down the bilirubin, an orange-yellow toxic waste product in her blood that made her skin turn yellow.

The hydrocephalic Collins baby also was doing well with hollow tubes implanted in his swollen brain draining off the fluids.

In the room down the hall, the Hernandez baby was dying. The one-month-old baby had a lethal genetic defect that would kill him before his first birthday, and there was nothing more that could be done.

The doctors tried to tell the parents this so they could prepare themselves for the sad inevitability, but the mother and father would not listen. They were going to take their baby home right away because they were convinced that witchcraft had caused the defect and that witchcraft could repair it.

Saddest of all was Baby Girl Jones. Something went wrong during birth and her blood did not get enough oxygen. Tests showed that she had suffered severe and irreversible brain damage.

Doctors could keep her alive for many months, if not years, with modern medical technology, but she never would be able to function on her own. The parents were told this, and after several days decided to let their daughter die. Nurses would continue to feed the baby and change her diapers, but they would give no drugs for the infection she had developed or do anything else that would prolong life.

Dr. Haggerty looked at the Jones baby for a moment and then moved on with her group following closely behind. There is usually little comment near the bedsides of babies beyond help because there's nothing much that can be done. It is particularly difficult for the nurses, however, because they feed, hug, and become attached to these babies, knowing that they are doomed.

□ □ □

Susan Loyd adjusted quickly to the hospital routine. Most of her time was either spent in the playroom with other children or being carted off by a nurse or aide for some test. Mark noticed that the jerking movements did not seem to be occurring as often as they had when Susan first arrived.

Dr. Ashbacher and Mark, who had spent his evenings reading about rheumatic disease and other conditions that caused chorea, were beginning to wonder if Susan had rheumatic disease at all.

The pediatrician who had referred Susan to Children's suspected rheumatic disease, and most of the doctors on the floor at first had agreed that this was most likely, but now the lab tests were all coming back normal.

Usually when bacteria invade an organism, the body fights back with biochemicals called antibodies, but the lab technicians could find no rheumatic disease antibodies in Susan's blood.

Also, all other blood tests were normal. And rheumatic disease is associated with heart trouble, but the cardiologist called in to check Susan could find nothing wrong.

As is so often the case in medicine, the negative findings did not completely rule out any particular disease but only made it less likely.

The books say that 72 percent of the muscle twitching known as chorea is caused by rheumatic disease, and in young girls the percentage is even higher. If rheumatic fever was not responsible for Susan's chorea, then what was? Perhaps the neurology department could explain it.

The neurologist arrived, gave Susan a special set of tests with a little rubber hammer and flashlight, and watched her when she had attacks. Finally he was satisfied.

Susan doesn't have chorea, he concluded. Chorea just doesn't look like that.

He suspected that it was nothing more than a nervous tick.

□ □ □

The next day, Mark and his classmate went to the well-baby clinic, where mothers bring their babies for routine checkups, an encounter much less threatening to the mothers and their babies than to the students who had never done it before.

After working for two straight weeks in wards where the children are so terribly sick and weak, it was jarring to see normal babies who would smile and cry and struggle when they were examined rather than lie there listless.

Well-baby clinic is much more typical of the type of work most pediatricians do than the wards on the floors above. Much of a pediatrician's time is spent assuring anxious mothers that everything is perfectly normal or that a given disease is self-limiting and will go away soon.

Pediatricians are experts in normal growth and as such differ sharply from their colleagues in adult medicine who know little about this. Pediatricians are forever measuring the mental and physical growth curves of their young patients against the established norm.

By three months babies should smile spontaneously and sit with their heads steady. By one year they should be able to drink from a cup, say three words other than "mama" and "dada" and walk backward. And by four years, they should be able to walk backward heel-to-toe, define words, and imitate the demonstrator. If they cannot do these things when they are supposed to, the pediatrician knows it is a sign of possible trouble that should be checked.

One of the jokes in medical circles is that students go into pediatrics because they do not want to deal with patients who are sick. Pediatricians do not concede that, but they do agree that a nice thing about the specialty is that they do not have to spend most of their time treating chronic disease.

Pull a child through a serious illness, they say, and he might have a chance for sixty more years of life. In adult medicine the physician is plagued with the frustration of being able to support his patient only through one chronic illness after another until one finally kills him.

In pediatrics, says Dr. Haggerty, there is the added reward of being able to help parents through those fearful moments when their child is sick and they do not know what it means. Sometimes one cannot do anything for the child, she said, but one can help the parents.

The bulletin boards in the wards are loaded with cards, letters, and snapshots from grateful parents.

One card came from the mother of a terminally ill leukemic. She wanted to thank the nurses and especially Dr. Haggerty, who spent the night sleeping on a cot in the ward next to her child. The nurses gave Dr. Haggerty the note. She still has it in her purse.

□ □ □

Susan's case was presented at an "attending rounds" conference, a one-hour session held four days a week to review the most interesting or complex cases handled by Dr. Haggerty's team.

Attending rounds can be a grueling experience for students and interns because the meeting is conducted by full-fledged faculty members who delight in testing their audience's knowledge with probing questions.

Consulting his notes as he went along, Mark slowly presented the data on Susan's case, speaking in a soft steady voice that betrayed none of the tension he was feeling.

Few questions were asked during the opening minutes of the presentation as pertinent data was written on the white blackboard with purple chalk by Dr. Karl Roth, a relaxed pipe-smoking expert in metabolic disease who had just started growing a beard.

Suddenly Dr. Roth stopped writing on the blackboard and turned to face Mark.

"She demonstrated the movements?" Dr. Roth said abruptly. "She has voluntary control?"

Hesitantly, Mark said she did. Dr. Roth turned back to the blackboard and wrote the word *voluntary,* putting a large star next to it.

Mark continued his presentation, but was immediately interrupted again. This time it was Dr. William Fox, the other attending on the team.

With long neatly combed hair, belled trousers, and a broad smile, the youthful Dr. Fox looked deceptively like a friendly Dr. Kildare. In fact, he was a hard-driving, challenging diagnostician who was forever pinning students and interns at the conference with difficult questions.

"Tell me more about the presenting complaint," Dr. Fox said, smiling at Mark. "Exactly what were the movements like? Why do you describe them as chorealike movements?"

Mark answered the questions, but Dr. Fox wanted more detail. Mark obviously was under a lot of pressure now, but his replies were quiet and to the point. When he did not know an answer he simply said he did not know, with neither excuses nor apologies.

Mark continued presenting more information for another twenty minutes, but the going was slow because he was constantly interrupted with questions. When he gave answers, other students and interns at the table were asked if they agreed and if not, why not.

"What were the pertinent negatives?" Dr. Fox asked, referring to negative findings that would rule out some problems.

The antibody studies and other blood tests were normal, Mark said, and the physical examination revealed nothing unusual. The family history offered no clues.

"All right, now, what do we have here?" Dr. Roth asked with his chalk ready. They had been going at it for almost an hour and Dr. Haggerty signaled him that time was running short.

One by one the students and interns offered possible explanations for Susan's problem, as Dr. Roth wrote them on the blackboard.

Contrary to popular belief, physicians rarely are able to make a conclusive diagnosis on the basis of one lab test or a physical exam.

The art of making a diagnosis is to aim for the most likely possibility without ruling out the less likely before the facts warrant it.

After ten minutes of discussion, Dr. Roth had written five broad categories that Susan's illness might fall within: (1) *neurological* (nerve-related), (2) *muscular,* (3) *tumor-* or *cancer-related,* (4) *psychosocial,* or (5) *rheumatic disease.*

The history and negative lab test almost eliminated the possibility of rheumatic disease, Dr. Roth said, putting a big *X* next to the words *rheumatic disease* he had written on the blackboard.

Muscular was also crossed out, because muscular diseases produce other problems in addition to twitching. The muscles feel abnormal upon examination. Often the child's muscles have wasted away.

Since the neurologist is an expert on neurological problems and could find no neurologic disease, Dr. Roth put an *X* next to that possibility, leaving only *tumor* and *psychosocial* as primary possibilities.

Dr. Roth tended to doubt "tumor" because there were no other findings to suggest this. A brain tumor, for instance, probably would produce a personality change or a neurologic problem like sharply narrowed vision.

They could give Susan an EMI scan, which was a new type of x-ray device that took several pictures of the brain at different levels, enabling a computer to reconstruct what amounted to a three-dimensional image.

But the x-ray procedure cost $250 for each picture and it would have been a waste of medical resources and the patient's time to do such a test unless there were stronger reasons for employing it. There are so many potential tests that can be done that a good physician orders only those he has reason to suspect might find something.

Some disease processes are subtle, and the first signs are just not clear enough to suggest anything certain to doctors. So they wait. Frequently the problem disappears and everything is fine. Sometimes the disease progresses, finally producing symptoms that suggest problems that can be checked out with a test. But this was not the case here.

Dr. Roth was particularly impressed with three findings—the absence of other symptoms and positive lab tests, the mother's preoccupation with her child's health, and the fact that Susan had voluntary control of the movements. Chorea is involuntary.

Pressing the chalk firmly against the blackboard, Dr. Roth underlined the word *psychosocial*.

Dr. Roth was convinced that Susan had a severe psychological problem. Psychologically caused twitching in a child this age is a particularly dangerous sign. Susan should be seen by a psychiatrist immediately.

Susan was released the next day after they contacted the referring pediatrician. He knew the family and wanted to discuss it with the parents himself. So they told Susan's mother only that the tests were normal and that their pediatrician would explain what had to be done now.

□ □ □

The final week of the pediatric rotation for Mark and his classmate was uneventful. They each had another admission. One of the babies on the ward went into cardiac arrest, and a code, calling for all available help, was announced over the public address system. A dozen doctors and nurses came running in from all over the place to resuscitate the child.

Mark and his classmate just missed it, though. They were down the hall running errands and by the time they got back the emergency team had brought the child back.

Baby Girl Marter had responded nicely to the blue light therapy during the week and would go home soon.

The Jones baby had not died yet, but was growing weaker.

Most of the other babies were doing satisfactorily.

Mark and his classmate ended their last week, said good-bye to the interns, residents, and nurses they had worked with, and left.

Next week they would start new rotations in other hospitals. And, in their place, other students would come to learn something about pediatrics.

17

Sweat streamed down Ron Gilliam's face, making it glisten in the dim light as he worked the set of drums clustered around him. The big room was packed tight with dancing bodies and spectators watching from the sides, but Ron was oblivious to them.

His mind was elsewhere, lost among the intricacies of rhythm and beat, anticipating the next moves of the other musicians. You could see he was in another world, the way he sat there with his head held erect, his back ramrod straight and his eyes seeing something no one else could see.

Ron was jamming with his friends, and it was a special occasion for him because this was his wedding reception. He played straight, without a break for more than two and a half hours. It was amazing, considering how sick he was.

Only the day before, Ron had been lying in a bed in the hemodialysis unit at the HUP having his blood cleansed by a kidney machine. He would be in the hospital again two days after his wedding, undergoing another seven-hour treatment.

While Ron played, Rikki mingled with the guests. A cluster of older women had come up from Rikki's home on Sea Island, South Carolina, sat in a circle in another room away from the blare of the music. Children ran around underfoot and people lined up to eat some of the eighty pounds of meat that Rikki's father, Vernon, a gourmet cook, had prepared.

But always Rikki would return to the room where people were dancing and sit down near the band, her head moving up and down with the beat, looking proud and beautiful in her floor-length rose velvet dress and green toga.

For the moment Rikki was thinking only of the party and the present, trying to forget the immediate past and the distant future that looked so bad for Ron.

□ □ □

A few days before the wedding, Dr. Grossman had contacted Rikki and Ron to give them the results of the tissue typing. The results were shockingly bad.

Probably because of blood-pressure pills Ron had been taking, his body had developed highly reactive antibodies. These are blood components that attack foreign matter such as bacteria and, unfortunately, transplanted kidneys.

The antibodies had been highly reactive in the test tube with samples from Ron's brother and other persons. Ordinarily this would have suggested that Ron's body would reject a kidney transplant, but this type of allergic condition was very rare.

Dr. Grossman thought it might have occurred only in the test tube and did not constitute a real threat to a kidney transplant. Still, it would have been too big a risk to justify Ron's brother's giving up one of his two kidneys.

Instead, a kidney from a cadaver would have to be used first. If it was rejected immediately, it would mean that Ron was doomed to use the machine for the rest of his life. If, on the other hand, his body rejected it only after several months or years, it would mean he was no more allergic than anyone else and it would be reasonable to chance a transplant from his brother. The best of all possibilities would be if the cadaver transplant showed signs of surviving indefinitely.

How long would it be before a cadaver kidney would be ready?

It was difficult to say. More than a hundred and fifty persons in the Philadelphia area were waiting for kidneys, and donations had been falling off to only a couple a month. Some patients had been waiting as long as three years. But Ron had a blood type that was easier to match a kidney with, so the wait should not be more than a couple of months.

Until then he and Rikki would have to wait, and three times a week Ron would go to the machine.

□ □ □

Ron's kidney condition had affected Rikki's professional life as well as her personal one. Not only had she become an expert on end-stage kidney disease, she was now also intensely studying the emotional effects of serious disease and medical management that psychologically disabled the patient.

Rikki was planning to write a technical paper on the stress of being on a kidney machine. And she had just finished a course on stress that discussed, among other things, how medical care itself could create a wound that often was more difficult to treat than the original affliction.

An obvious example of this was the kidney-machine patient who was burdened by the psychological stress of total dependency on a machine that, while it kept him alive, constantly reminded him how close death was.

Though the machine had kept Ron alive, his life was far from satisfactory. Unable to travel, he could not make concert tours, and the contacts he had been building in New York had faded. He got a job with a band, but was fired when the other players saw the needle marks on his arm. They mistook his wounds from the dialysis-machine needles for the signs of drug addiction.

Why didn't he tell them he was a kidney patient?

"They don't want sick people either," he said.

Before his illness, he had been playing several times a week. Now he was lucky if he got one or two gigs a month.

It felt good to be married after all the indecision prompted by the disease and the question of whether or not Ron would go on the machine. It gave the young couple some sense of control. They had made a joint decision. That had combined their lives. They had made a formal commitment to confront this thing as a couple. And also they would share the joys.

But it was a *ménage à trois,* the machine being the third member of the household. Rikki would tell the people close to her: "That machine is a part of my mind now. Just as I have admitted Ronny to my mind, I have admitted the machine. It's a part of my thinking. It's just as real to me," she would say holding up her left hand, "as this wedding ring."

18

It was a typical busy morning on the fourth floor of the HUP, and most of the twenty-two operating rooms were in use. The masked surgeons and nurses could be seen in each operating room through the windows of the swinging doors, crowding around patients covered by green surgical drapes.

Dr. Cletus W. Schwegman was in Operating Room Five, exploring the abdomen of a fifty-year-old man to find out if he had intestinal cancer.

Next door, in Operating Room Six, Dr. Julius A. Mackie was doing a breast biopsy on a thirty-nine-year-old woman who probably didn't have cancer but they couldn't be sure without the operation.

And down the hall at the other end of the building, Dr. Horace MacVaugh III was well into his second open-heart operation of the day.

In the hallways outside the operating rooms, patients were lying on litters in various levels of consciousness, having been mildly sedated before they were brought there. Soon it would be their time and they would be wheeled into one of the rooms where they would be greeted by an anesthesiologist who would prepare them for the surgeon.

For four weeks, the second-year students taking Surgery 200 would spend their mornings in this world. They would hold clamps, cut sutures and perhaps help sew a wound shut, but nothing much more complicated than that.

In so short a period, they couldn't even begin to learn surgery, but at least the introductory course would give them an idea of what surgery could and could not do.

□ □ □

To most people, surgery is the most dramatic of medical specialties and the operating room is an awesome place where life hangs by a thread and the slightest mistake by the surgeon means death.

In reality, such high drama is unusual and, as the students would soon learn, the mood of the operating room is determined more by the personality of the surgeon than the condition of the patient.

In no other specialty of medicine is the star system more evident than in surgery. In his operating room, the senior surgeon is boss and he is the one who sets the tone and pace. Even the procedures designed to maintain sterile conditions tend to elevate him like the rituals in a royal court.

The surgeon enters the operating room after everything has been made ready, his freshly scrubbed hands held in front of him, and immediately all tend to his needs. A sterile surgical pack containing towels to dry his still wet hands and a robe to wear lie open, waiting for only him or his aides to touch. The scrub nurse helps him pull on his rubber gloves while the circulating nurse ties his sterile surgical robe from the back. This completed, all those standing around the operating table draw back and make a path for him as though out of respect, but in reality to keep from contaminating his hands or gown.

The hierarchy is a very real thing in surgery. The senior men, and they are all men, get first choice of the operating rooms, and when someone has to be bumped from the schedule because of an emergency or lack of space, it is always the junior surgeon who has to tell his patient that he must wait another day.

On top of this hierarchy at Penn was Dr. Johnathan E. Rhoads. He had so much prestige that he stood by himself in the estimation of the residents under him.

Asked why he was so highly regarded, two residents snapped back almost in unison: "Because he's a great man." He was nationally known for the many research papers he had published, the men he had trained and the medical groups he had headed. Out of respect for his position, it was always the chief resident who assisted Dr. Rhoads in the operating room.

They referred to him as "the old man" or "J.E.R." or, when he was not in earshot, simply as "Johnathan." Everyone knew what "Johnathan" they meant by the way the name was pronounced.

□ □ □

In Operating Room Five this morning, Dr. Schwegman was being helped by Dr. Richard Spence, a friendly good-natured resident, and Mrs. Judy Aronchick, a University of Pennsylvania psychology graduate and now a second-year medical student. Standing on a platform to give her a better angle, she held on to retractors that kept the surgical wound open so Dr. Schwegman could operate.

The surgical drapes that covered the patient and the surgical gowns the nurses and doctors wore were green because under the bright operating lights the traditional hospital white made a glare that was hard on the eyes.

The only one in the room who didn't wear green that morning was Joan Johnson, who wore the pink uniform of another department.

On the fourth floor Ms. Johnson was known as the cancer lady because it was her job to collect samples of cancerous tissue for a research project that was under way. Whenever you saw her pink uniform in an operating room, you knew there was a good chance that the patient had cancer.

"Yeah, there it is," Dr. Schwegman said, his hand inside the cavity of the man's abdomen. The nurse slapped a scalpel into his other outstretched hand; he worked some more and then pulled out a lump of tissue he had just cut loose.

"Gentlemen," he said, holding the tissue up, "that's a carcinoma. You can feel it."

A laboratory study would have to be done to confirm that it was cancer, as Dr. Schwegman suspected, but there was no doubt in his mind because he had seen too much of it before. Within minutes the specimen was on its way to the pathology laboratory, carried in a green towel by pathology resident Dr. Albert Keshgegian, who had been summoned to the operating room.

Dr. Keshgegian would freeze the specimen in liquid nitrogen, a hair-thin piece of the tissue would be sliced off and stained, and a pathologist would study it under the microscope. It would take about ten minutes. Meanwhile, everyone in Operating Room Five would wait.

□ □ □

Dr. Schwegman ran a somewhat formal though not tense operating room. He was known for being fast, which was highly regarded, and for starting early in the morning. Being a senior surgeon with stature in the hierarchy, the nursing and anesthesiology departments accommodated him even though he started surgery at 7:30, a half hour before anyone else.

The operating room of Dr. William T. Fitts, Jr., who had been department chairman but gave it up because he preferred surgery to paper work, had a friendly, homespun air to it. He was one of the few surgeons to wear a sweatband on his forehead, and he was forever prodding his students and residents with questions as he worked.

Wearing a fiber optic light like a miner's lamp for better visibility, Dr. MacVaugh directed his operations like the captain on the bridge of a ship, giving orders to assistants and the technicians running the heart-lung machine that kept his open-heart patients alive.

No other surgeon at Penn was as busy as Dr. MacVaugh, who did up to sixty operations a month, nor did any other doctor better illustrate the classic personality of a surgeon.

He was an aggressive, decisive, athletic man who was not easily rattled or given to pensive contemplation. He played excellent golf, flew his own plane, and almost became an astronaut, but decided against it at the last moment because it would have taken him away from surgery too long.

Surgeons are doers, almost compulsive people, who are attracted to this specialty because it is a field of medicine in which action is swift and the results, whether they are good or bad, are quickly apparent. Surgeons are forever chiding their colleagues in internal medicine for spending hours upon hours diagnosing obscure diseases they can do nothing about.

There is a joke in medical circles: Internists know everything but can do nothing, while surgeons know nothing, but do everything. It is an exaggeration, of course, but there is little time for brooding or contemplation in the operating room.

What brooder could stand at the side of the operating table every weekday morning as Dr. MacVaugh did, stare down at the exposed and throbbing human heart, and then cut into it to make repairs?

□ □ □

Dr. Keshgegian returned with a piece of paper in his hand. "Dr. Schwegman," he announced the moment he walked into the room, "it's an adenocarcinoma."

Dr. Schwegman nodded his thanks and started up the operation again, Dr. Keshgegian left and the cancer lady packed up her sample of tissue for the research laboratory. The laboratory would use the tissue to produce an experimental vaccinelike substance that might help the patient fight the cancer should it start up again.

□ □ □

The surgeon's day was a long one, especially for the house staff and the students. It began at 7:00 A.M., when the hospital was still mostly asleep and the hallways were empty.

For the most part, the only sign of life was the smell of coffee coming from the staff cafeteria. It was taken over at this hour by teams of surgical residents, interns, and students going over the status of all patients on their service before the morning operations began.

The discussion was called dry rounds because the doctors sat at a table instead of going from patient to patient. And they didn't talk of disease processes so much as they did about the minutia of preoperative and postoperative care. They spoke of changing sumps and drains, fluid input and urine output, temperatures and pain medication.

It was not a particularly challenging part of their job, but the surgical house staff spent much of the morning and all of the afternoon attending to such details, writing everything they did onto charts and chasing after lab reports and x-ray studies by telephone or on foot.

And the evenings were spent providing postoperative care or seeing that everything was in readiness for the surgery scheduled for the next day. In many respects it was a tedious matter of solving thousands of little problems.

Interspersed among these activities were lectures held daily for the students and periodic conferences like the monthly morbidity and mortality review, which everyone attended, including the house staff and senior surgeons.

The purpose of these reviews was to find ways to improve techniques and identify mistakes so that they would not be repeated.

The mortality rate for general surgery in an institution like the HUP ranged from between 1 and 1.5 percent. Since the general surgeons did about five hundred cases a month at Penn, that came to about seven deaths to be considered at these conferences.

Most of the deaths involved high-risk patients. It was unusual for a patient to die unexpectedly from an unanticipated cause, but a busy general surgeon would run into this on the average of once every two years.

When the students were not attending conferences or lectures in the afternoon, they followed their intern or resident, rushing from room to room and floor to floor to tend the surgical wounds of patients already operated on and prepare others for the surgery to come.

This was when the house staff got to know something about the patients, especially if the resident was gregarious and liked to talk while he worked over the patient, changing bandages and drainage tubes. There were so many patients:

There was the Ecker boy in 1603. Surgeons had to take most of his intestines, which had been destroyed by disease, and he would have to be fed by tube for the rest of his life.

Mrs. Burns was still complaining about the lemonade being bitter and demanding more pain drugs. And next door Billings was terrified about the colostomy he would get tomorrow morning.

The most cheerful person on the sixth floor was Mrs. Talbot, a huge woman who was five feet nine inches tall and weighed 310 pounds.

For twenty-eight years she had tried to lose weight with all types of diets and programs. She would lose forty or fifty pounds, but then gain it back. So now she was in the hospital, waiting for an operation to solve her problem.

Dr. Ernest F. Rosato would bring her to the operating room and tie off most of her small intestine, through which the body absorbs food. Afterward she would have to go to the toilet four or five times a day, but if she was typical, she would also lose a hundred pounds in the next eighteen months.

Most of the patients were glad when the residents and students came by. It was a chance to break the monotony or grab a bit of information with a quick question.

But some patients would just lie in bed, immersed in their silent fears or depressions, indifferent to the ministrations of doctors who could do something for them but just not enough.

□ □ □

So much of general surgery deals with cancer and so often cancer cannot be surgically cured. It would be an overwhelmingly sad business for a poet or someone else who dwells on the human plight, but surgeons tend not to be such people.

They think of the present and in terms of what can be done. If it can be done, they do it: Cut out the cancer and cure the patient. If it can't be done, it can't be done, and they accept that. As they see it, it's not their fault.

Some students were not ready to accept this resignation. This being their first direct contact with surgery, many were seeing patients die for the first time, and death and pain to them was still very much a personal thing. If death could not be prevented, they felt, then it should at least be treated with the reverence of sadness.

In the coming years, as these students moved through school and the different clinical rotations, they would each deal with this problem on their own terms.

Some would use denial and simply not think about it in personal terms. Some would avoid the issue by going into specialties in which it was not such a problem, like ophthalmology, dermatology, or research that did not involve dealing with patients at all. And still others would work their feelings through and become better physicians for having done so.

19

The thin, toothless old man with gray stubble on his chin strained to lift his head up from the operating table so he could watch the surgeons preparing his left leg for the operation. Disease had cut off the blood supply to the limb and it was permanently frozen in a bent position. Soon the anesthesiologist would put the man to sleep. When he woke up the leg would be gone.

Medical students Daniel Merges and John Stefano watched from the side as a surgical resident reviewed the medical and social history quietly so the patient couldn't hear. Both students were gowned and masked. Later, John would scrub and assist in the amputation.

The old man looked more resigned than scared or sad, like someone who had come to accept life's bad fortunes, of which there had been many for him. He had neither money nor relatives and it was not clear when he would be able to leave Philadelphia General Hospital (PGH) because the disease had already claimed his right leg. It had been amputated a year earlier.

The old man had been living with some other men in a room over a store, but with no legs he'd be too much of a burden to his roommates. He would have to make other arrangements. For the moment, however, there was nowhere else he could go, so he would stay at PGH for a few weeks. Or months. Or maybe a year or so.

The operation didn't take long. Slicing through the tissue layer by layer, tying off blood vessels as they went, the surgeons quickly reached the white bone, cut through it with a serrated wire attached to two handles, and closed the stump with a few strong stitches. Soon the man was back in the fourth floor men's ward where he would begin his long recuperation.

□ □ □

Even on the first day, it was obvious to the students that the types of patients and medical and social problems at a city-owned hospital like PGH were strikingly different from those found at HUP, only a half block away.

PGH was a unique hospital in Philadelphia. It was unique because it never turned anyone away and, as a result, got all the patients the other hospitals didn't want.

It admitted the patients who had no money or insurance. It accepted the senile and the alcoholics and the drug addicts and the prisoners. It accepted the patients with chronic problems that would outlive their insurance benefits and provided a home for people who had no other place to go once they had been treated.

Thus, not only did PGH give the indigent and old in the city a court of last resort, it offered medical students a unique opportunity to see diseases that had advanced to a late and frequently fatal stage, because the poor were slower to get medical care than the more affluent.

Before the class of '78 graduated, the historic city hospital would be closed by a city administration that did not give medical care of the poor a high priority. It would not be as tragic as some had predicted, however. Because the poor were now being covered by state and federal medical insurance, they would be accepted by nearby hospitals that were confident they would get paid.

The undesirable patients, like the alcoholics and senile, would be farmed out and reluctantly accepted since there was no more PGH to warehouse them in and calm the conscience of society. And those who were simply old would be sent to a nursing home the city would open up, a more economical and desirable place for such patients anyhow.

The three second-year students assigned to the PGH surgical service on this particular month were:

John Stefano, twenty-three, Penn pre-med graduate, who had gotten married three weeks before medical school started the year before.

Daniel Merges, twenty-three, a Notre Dame biology graduate, who planned to marry in June.

And Jeffrey Rubinstein, twenty-two, a Bucknell University biology graduate who was about to become engaged.

□ □ □

By modern hospital standards that called for only two patients to a room, the wards at PGH were huge, with thirteen beds down one wall and thirteen more down the other. In front of each bed was an easy chair with wooden arms. The patients spent most of their days sitting in these chairs, lined up like so many passengers in a bus going nowhere. At mealtimes, aides placed trays across the arms of the chairs, which then became the patients' dining room.

Each morning a white cloud billowed into the ward. A half dozen or so interns, residents, and students in their white coats went down one side and then back up the other reviewing the status of the patients. And as the cloud passed the beds and chairs, some of the patients called out, while others continued to mumble whatever they had happened to be mumbling all morning to no one in particular:

"Where's my doctor? Where's my doctor? Are you my doctor?" a thin, old woman yelled at John Stefano, who left the disappearing cloud of doctors for a moment. He told the woman that he wasn't her doctor, but that he'd check around for her.

A few chairs away another woman was talking to herself, repeating the same phrases over and over.

"The coffee was delicious. Please remove the tray. The coffee was delicious. Please remove the tray. The coffee was . . ."

Surgical rounds in all hospitals are disturbingly fast, if not abrupt, but they were particularly quick at PGH because so many of the patients were not sick and hence didn't take up the doctors' time during rounds.

These were the "disposition problems," or "dispos" as they were referred to in PGH parlance. They were the patients who were there and whose cases could not be closed only because there was nowhere else for them to go.

One woman on the floor had been there for almost two years. Her husband visited her three times a week, but refused to take her home, claiming that he was too sick to take care of her even though she would require only minor attention.

On a typical day this month, twenty-five of the forty-one women in the surgical ward were disposition problems, which was about average at PGH. Many of them weren't even very sick when they came to the emergency room for some minor illness, but were admitted anyway because the doctors were afraid they'd die of malnutrition or neglect if they were sent away, they were so frail and old.

□ □ □

As the days passed and the students moved through their term at PGH, they learned as much about themselves and the ills of society as they did about the physical problems of their patients. In many unexpected ways they were tested, and on some occasions found themselves lacking or at least they thought they were lacking.

One student was disturbed because of how he came to feel about an angry, seventy-two-year-old woman who would fight with the doctors and students whenever they came near. She would tear the intravenous tubes out of her arms and would scream when anyone touched her. After a while the students began to lose interest in her and disliked caring for her.

Another student was disappointed with himself because after a couple of weeks he found he could walk by the woman who was always calling out for a doctor and ignore her. It didn't help his conscience to know that the woman always yelled for help when someone in a white coat walked by, even though nothing was troubling her.

These disturbing self-discoveries were made at all the hospitals the

Surgery 200 students rotated through, not just at PGH.

Sometimes residents referred to difficult patients in unbecoming ways when discussing them privately in the doctors' lounge or staff cafeteria. Comatose patients were called gorks and troublesome, demanding patients were toads. Failing patients were said to be "going down the tube," and when the ailing died, they "went to China."

These expressions were frequently heard at HUP and PGH and the other hospitals. The Surgery 200 students at first didn't like this, but after a while many found themselves using the same expressions, much to their disappointments.

Many of the students worried about this, afraid they would become hardened, and they talked among themselves about ways to avoid it.

It didn't bother the residents to know that students thought some of them harsh or unfeeling with their patients. The residents had been students themselves only a few years ago and at that time felt as these students did. But the residents changed, just as they knew that today's students would change.

Said one of the residents:

"You don't cross that line that separates doctors from the rest of the world until you become an intern and have the responsibility for the patient. You build defenses. Even with the defenses, when the patient begins to fail or dies, you go home and you're uncertain, not knowing if you shouldn't have done something differently because he was your patient, your responsibility. Students don't have any responsibilities. They don't need the defense yet."

The sick and old and dying—such images in any hospital are so powerful and moving that no one can confront them day after day without some protective mechanism. It was particularly difficult at a hospital like PGH, where illness was compounded by the devastations of poverty, senility, alcoholism, and social neglect.

John Stefano was particularly moved, and disturbed, by one dying old woman. No one ever came to see her, and he couldn't understand why she had been abandoned. Her hands were wrinkled and thin and they reminded him of the hands of his grandmother, who had died recently.

"It was very difficult for me to understand," John said, "because my family is very Italian and they take care of each other. Like my grandmother, when she was dying, everyone in the family responded . . . there was always someone visiting . . . her death was like a family affair. But this old woman, no one comes to see her. It's hard to understand why the people she took care of all her life aren't here taking care of her now."

He paused and looked down at a piece of loose thread he had been nervously playing with on his white coat. Then he looked up again.

"Some of the people are just left here to die," he said, his voice trailing off.

Just about all of the students agreed that they had been changed by the weeks they spent at PGH, HUP, Presbyterian, Graduate, and the other hospitals affiliated with Penn. They knew they were not quite the same people they had been before they started the rotations. But they didn't know how they changed or even what happened during those eight weeks to effect the change, small as it might have been.

It was no one thing. It was many fleeting moments, images that flashed before them so quickly they weren't aware of them until hours later or maybe that night when they were talking to their wives or other students.

* The old man was dying. He had advanced lung cancer that had spread throughout his body. He lay in his bed in the surgical intensive-care unit, struggling to breathe with a plastic face mask while a surgeon and another doctor argued whether he belonged in the surgical intensive-care unit or the medical unit. The case was hopeless and neither wanted him.

* The old woman was so grateful because the residents and students had done so much for her. She wanted to repay them for their kindness, she wanted to give them money, but the students refused, saying it wasn't necessary.

* The disposition problem patients were so happy that the two students were taking the time to talk to them and to get to know them a little bit. The regular doctors had too many other things that had to be done to take time for such things. One woman was so delighted, she wouldn't let the students go until they let her kiss their hands.

* The old former farmhand from the South was diabetic, blind, and had no legs. Frequently at night he got confused and yelled out to the nurses: "Please, please put me back on my horse. Put me back on my horse."

* The women from Jewish Family Services came in to visit the patients and make them feel less deserted. The kindly women looked so out of place with their fine clothes and Gucci handbags and big smiles in a place where so many people never smiled. A white-haired old lady with her hospital gown opened at the back walked up to one of them and mumbled something. "Yes, yes, yes," the well-dressed woman said brightly. "But we've got to make the best of what we've got." The old lady nodded and went back to her chair to consider the advice.

* The thirty-five-year-old schizophrenic wandered around a city park for weeks, his legs wet, dirty, and infected. Finally the legs became gangrenous and he could wander no more. Police brought him in and the surgeons took both legs.

□ □ □

The students finished Surgery 200 with mixed feelings. They were impressed by the marvelous things surgeons were capable of doing, but by and large they didn't think much of surgery as a specialty.

They saw surgeons as a rushed, impersonal bunch who didn't have rapport with their patients. They found most of the work tedious, without intellectual excitement—esoteric craftsmanship with a lot of time being wasted chasing after lab reports, x-ray studies, and medical aides who failed to do things they were supposed to do.

They didn't like the abrupt, episodic nature of surgery, where the surgeon would meet, operate on, and discharge a patient all in a few weeks, never to see him again.

Most of the students wanted to be primary physicians who were interested in their patients and their families. They wanted longer, more personal contact, something that wasn't seen very often during the eight weeks of their experiences in surgery.

Listening to the students talking about the disappointment with surgery, surgical intern Dr. Arnold Meshkov nodded knowingly.

"Yeah, that's the way I felt up until my last year in school. I wanted to be in medicine, but by the end of my third year I was tired of these endless discussions about diseases no one could do anything about. I wanted to get into an area of medicine where you could do something positive. That's when I decided to go into surgery."

20

It was late at night and Marge Shamonsky was sitting with two interns in the almost empty staff cafeteria at the HUP. For nearly twenty minutes the interns had been talking about medicine, other house staff officers, and academic politics. They had paid no attention to Marge.

Marge tended to be a quiet and shy woman, but periodically she would gird herself and ask a question in an attempt to participate. The interns would respond, but the answers were curt, and immediately they would resume their private conversation, returning Marge to the role of silent observer.

The second year of medical school had not been going well for Marge. She had been unable to find camaraderie in the hospitals.

Her first rotation three months earlier had been a surprise and a disappointment. It was one of the two major rotations—Surgery 200. There was no personal contact. The attendings and other physicians seemed indifferent to the students and teaching. And worst of all, she felt she was being ignored by everyone. Slowly Marge was coming to hate going to the hospital each day.

Things improved when she moved on to her next rotation in psychiatry. She liked talking about the mind and people's emotions and fears and a lot of the other things that were never considered elsewhere in the hospital. For a while she thought of becoming a psychiatrist, but Freudian analysis turned her off.

She started her Medicine 200 rotation with the hope, if not expectation, that things would improve, but instead they got worse. The intern she was assigned to was very knowledgeable about medicine, but he was one of the coldest persons Marge had ever met.

"He won't even say hello to me when I come in in the morning," Marge said, complaining to Randy one night at home at the start of the rotation.

Randy looked up from his textbook and nodded. He understood what Marge was talking about because he had seen it himself. He'd experienced it himself. Big hospitals and big cities were too impersonal for him and it was clear that his new wife joined him in these feelings.

Marge sat down at the kitchen table with Randy and sighed. "Randy," she said evenly, "he won't even acknowledge my presence. When I ask him questions he talks to me in an angry tone, almost a disgusted way."

Marge came to realize how impersonal medicine could be a few days later when a terminally ill patient she was helping to take care of died. It was the first death of her young career and she was very disappointed with the way her intern had handled it.

Over the weeks Marge had come to know the woman and her family fairly well. The woman had aplastic anemia and everyone knew it would only be a matter of time. Marge spoke at length to her patient and the relatives, and a nice relationship developed.

Marge and her intern were on another floor when the call from the nurse came. The woman had died. The relatives wanted to talk to someone. The intern was outraged by the intrusion and forbade it. He was busy taking care of sick people who were still alive and these people wanted to talk about a patient who was dead. Nothing could be done for her now.

Marge was so depressed by the incident that she wanted to talk to someone about it. But there was no one to talk to. Randy was out that night doing his own rotation and Marge didn't feel comfortable discussing such things with other students or anyone on the house staff. It was simply not the thing to do. It wasn't cool. And the house staff and attendings rarely had time to adequately explain medicine and technology, let alone something like this—emotions—which they seemed to think unimportant. Marge was beginning to wonder if it was unprofessional to have emotions.

She wished she could talk about a lot of things with her new husband. But there was so little time, what with both of them in different hospitals on different rotations. There were so many night calls. And weekend work. Their marriage was new. They still didn't know each other that well. And many things still had to be worked out. The new marriage and getting to know someone she had met only a year earlier was a stress in Marge's life.

And the impersonal hospitals and the rotations were another stress. It was hard to get to know people because every month the students would switch to a new rotation in a different hospital with different people. It was like starting her life all over again every four weeks, with no chance to develop anything that was lasting, personal, and caring.

Slowly the fearful thought started to evolve.

Maybe, Marge wondered, she wasn't really the kind of person who should become a physician. Maybe she should leave medical school.

□ □ □

Few of the other students in the class of '78 seriously considered leaving. But many shared Marge's disappointment over the impersonality of everything. And some realized almost immediately that they were going to have to change their career plans. They discovered that their expectations for a particular specialty were romantic or unrealistic for their type of personality.

Only one rotation during the summer in the cancer wards of Harvard's Peter Bent Brigham Hospital in Boston convinced Barbara that she did not, as she had always thought, want to go into clinical cancer research. She had seen too many terminal cases that summer, and young people slowly dying, to feel comfortable about working in a specialty like oncology. She remembered one patient from South America, a very friendly man with a wry sense of humor. She had been following him as her patient for two weeks. One morning she came in and talked with him for a bit. That afternoon she saw the pathologists dissecting his body on the autopsy table.

Kate Treadway and Jim Nestor also quickly changed their career plans. They had both wanted to go into pediatrics, but after taking Pediatrics 200 they knew that caring for sick children wasn't for them.

As a former teacher of six- to nine-year-olds, Kate was accustomed to taking her time, slowly building up a relationship with her students. But in pediatrics there wasn't time for this. The contact was intense, but too brief to be anything but superficial, she thought, and she didn't like it. She started thinking of a career in internal medicine.

Jim didn't like to see sick kids. Children had always been cute puppies to him, something to play with and laugh with. But at Children's Hospital the children were really sick, and many of them were too ill even to talk or relate. It was too depressing.

Also Jim had had a bad experience as a student. The attendings and house staff tended to reassure him when he asked them how he was doing. Then in the end they gave him a poor evaluation. He thought it was dishonest. It happened on one of his first hospital rotations and immediately made him wary of any further dealings with attendings or residents. No, he didn't want pediatrics. He would have to find something else.

The clinical work was getting to Matt. He loved surgery and spent every moment he could in the operating rooms, but he was driving himself too hard with too few emotional rewards. Periodically broody, he would often escape by himself and ponder his insecurity before returning to the hospital again with a vengeance to do more and harder and better work.

Rikki Lights was disappointed because she hadn't found the art of medicine. She had expected an art—a creativity—to this profession, but so far she could find nothing creative at all.

It was just a matter of doing a lot of mundane things in the hospital and watching other people doing a lot of mundane things—drawing blood and filling out medical charts and chasing after technicians to get lab results, and spending hour after hour on the telephone. Where was the creativity of pondering information, she wondered, and putting it together in a creative way to arrive at a diagnosis or deduce new information.

Mark Reber, who at thirty was older than the average second-year student, was discovering that his maturity and ability to relate warmly to patients was not very highly valued by most house staff officers.

Having worked with mentally disabled children, Mark had developed the ability to quickly establish a sensitive rapport with the people he dealt with, especially children. He had always thought that this would be a valuable asset for a physician, but no one took notice of his abilities.

Instead the attendings and residents seemed far more impressed by the information that the students could provide or the journal references they could quote or other intellectual attainments. It was a disappointment, and Mark wondered if this was why medicine was so often criticized by patients as being impersonal. Mark wondered if the system would tend to make sensitive people harder and insensitive.

Many black students had come to the hospital rotations looking for examples of discrimination against black patients, but they found little of it. The discrimination that did exist consisted of ward patients being treated with less personal rapport than the patients with private physicians. It just happened that more patients without money were black than white. The students found it difficult to accept the uncaring treatment of ward patients as a necessary expedient in a teaching institution.

Richard Ellison, a black student from New York City, was particularly disturbed by the way white interns and residents used black ward patients to learn how to practice medicine and then, when they knew how, went into private practice and served almost all-white populations, leaving the black ghettos without physicians. He did not think that the ward patients received a lower quality of care than did private patients. But he did think that the interchange between physicians and ward patients was more brusque.

Conrad King, another black student, thought the ward patients were subjected to a lot more examinations and tests than private patients. Labored over by inexperienced students, the ward patients got "million-dollar" workups, more for educational purposes than for the patients' needs. The house staff wouldn't think of subjecting private patients to so many tests, because they have guardian angels in the form of their attending physicians.

The students were learning a lot as they moved through their first year in the hospital. And a lot of what they were learning had more to do with society and themselves as people than it did with the practice of medicine.

Their attitudes would change in later years as they became more sophisticated and the initial shock of seeing so much in such a short period had passed.

But not all of the disappointment would go away.

21

The new patients being admitted to the HUP medical service started arriving on the floors at about lunchtime. One of the patients was Robert Zinbar, an affable, forty-year-old insurance salesman who didn't think he had anything seriously wrong with him.

At first Mr. Zinbar resisted the counsel of his personal physician to go into the HUP to have it checked out. It was such a minor thing. He had cut his hand on his mowing machine. The family physician treated the wound but it refused to heal. Mr. Zinbar's physician agreed that it was probably nothing serious. "But why take a chance when you don't have to?" Mr. Zinbar remembered his doctor telling him. "Isn't that what you always tell your customers when you're selling them insurance?" the doctor chided him. So to humor his friend and physician, Mr. Zinbar checked into the HUP.

Shortly after coming into the hospital, Marianna Pavsek, a twenty-two-year-old second-year student with long brown hair, deep dark eyes, and a very gentle manner, took several vials of blood from Mr. Zinbar. Marianna put the blood into rubber-stoppered tubes, labeled them with Mr. Zinbar's name, and took them up to the laboratory.

Mr. Zinbar would undergo a battery of x-ray examinations and other lab tests. He would spend hours giving his medical history to Marianna, the medical resident, and later a hematologist who specialized in cancer of the blood. But the explanation of Mr. Zinbar's problem, the reason why his wound had failed to heal, was contained in the vials of blood Marianna had drawn shortly after he arrived.

□ □ □

Considering how far science has advanced in recent years, it is surprising that so much of what a medical student learns still comes from that old educational standby, apprenticeship training acquired at the side of the journeyman physician.

More than half of the four years in medical school is spent at bedside. Students may get the basic information and general principles from books and lectures. But it is on the wards, by the bedsides, that they learn the nuts and bolts of becoming a doctor—the symbolic, almost ritualistic, things like taking blood pressure, looking down the throat for infection, listening to the heart with a stethoscope, feeling for an enlarged liver, drawing a blood sample.

Part of their education on the wards comes from dealing with patients and their varied problems—patients who are poor, or sick or scared, or dying. Another part comes from seeking the approval of their peers and trying to emulate the doctors.

It is impossible to assess the effect that these things have on the students; it cannot be measured the way performance on a pathology or physiology quiz is scored. But such things are very much part of the making of a doctor, both in the best and in the worst senses of the word.

Suitable role models are very important to medical students. These are the physicians the students can look up to and emulate, not only in the way they perform technically but in the way they act as human beings—the way they deal with patients, peers, and subordinates.

The students see how their role model integrates his personal life and ideals into his professional life. In a very subtle way, the role model's actions help shape the student's professional identity. But the model reinforces rather than changes the student because the student tends to gravitate toward physicians who are somewhat like himself in manner, principles, and personality. Hence a highly competitive student like Matt Lotysh might look to cardiovascular surgeon Dr. Horace MacVaugh III, the most controversial and productive surgeon at the HUP, a flier and an athlete. Whereas Mark Reber would gravitate toward someone like Dr. Rosalind Y. Ting, an extremely gentle, socially concerned, developmental pediatrician from China, who worked at Children's Hospital.

Most academic physicians at a place like Penn tended to be conservative in dress, liberal in politics, affluent in manner, and generally reserved. But there were exceptions—like the outrageous Dr. James E. Nixon, an iconoclastic orthopedic surgeon at Graduate Hospital, and Dr. Gunter Haase, a cultured and dignified neurologist at Pennsylvania Hospital, who spoke with a German accent, skied in Europe, and looked something like a character out of a Monte Carlo casino scene in a James Bond movie.

Role models are so important that the students' most frequent criticism of Penn as a teaching institution would be the lack of black and women role models. Neither was frequently encountered among the ranks of house officers or attending physicians at the HUP.

□ □ □

Dr. Malcolm Cox was almost a caricature of the bright, sophisticated, always-on-top-of-it, Penn medical department house officer, an image enhanced by his tall slender physique, perfectly proper mustache, and the

British accent he acquired in his native South Africa. Quiet-spoken and always in control, he invariably carried a collapsible pointer with him to indicate interesting things on x-ray films. As the chief medical resident at the HUP, he was the highest-ranking physician on the medical house staff, which was composed of sixty-three interns and residents in the medical department.

The competition for this job at a place like the HUP was vigorous, and the winner was considered among the best of the young doctors coming into medicine. Ambitious students were well advised to study carefully the way such successful people handled themselves on rounds.

On this particular rotation, Dr. Cox headed a team that included Marianna, whom everyone called Nana, another second-year student, Michael Rosen, and two interns, Drs. Gene Lugano and Paul Goldberg.

On selected mornings, Mike and Nana would follow Dr. Cox and the other members of his team on attending rounds, an educational and patient-care ritual in which Dr. Cox would pass on some of his wisdom.

After spending an hour or two discussing new cases, the team would visit the patients in their rooms. And while the responsible nurse hovered in the background ready to answer questions or prod the doctors into writing a needed order, the swarm of white coats would engulf each patient in turn.

"I can't rest. I'm so scared."

The voice came from an almost blind, white-haired old woman whose face was buried in her pillow. Reaching out with thin fingers, she felt the arm of Dr. Cox, who stood near her bed.

"What are you afraid of?" the tall Dr. Cox asked, bending down so they could hear each other. The woman had just been transferred from another hospital where she had had a colon operation.

"What are you afraid of?" Dr. Cox repeated.

At first the woman said nothing. But then through the pillow, which muffled the words, Dr. Cox could hear: "Of the unknown."

Dr. Cox touched her. "There's nothing here that's unknown," Dr. Cox said. He told her that they knew pretty much what was wrong with her, but that some tests had to be done.

"I'm going to ask God that you're honest with me," she said, feeling her way up Dr. Cox's arm with her fingers.

"Please trust us," Dr. Cox said.

The woman was disoriented, having been suddenly transferred from one hospital to another after surgery and unable to see. The team left her and went down the hall to another room and another patient.

"It's a classical stimulus withdrawal situation," Dr. Cox said in answer to a question from one of those in his retinue.

□ □ □

The laboratory technician came into the office of pathologist Dr. Hugh Bonner with some microscope slides. It was her job to screen blood smears taken from hospital patients, and whenever something unusual showed up she would bring it to Dr. Bonner's attention. These samples were from Mr. Zinbar.

Dr. Bonner put the slide under the microscope and focused it. A field with the red dots of hundreds of blood cells came into sharp view. It did not look normal. Instead of being evenly scattered, many of the red cells were piled on top of one another in what is called a rouleaux formation.

Very prominent in the field of red cells were huge plasma cells stained blue. They had big off-center purple nuclei. And the little platelets, responsible for coagulating the blood, were fewer in number than normal in this sample.

The disease process was so obvious that the one blood sample was almost enough to make a definite diagnosis. Robert Zinbar had multiple myeloma. This is a cancer of the bone marrow in which components of the blood are produced.

Usually a bone marrow tap is necessary to prove the diagnosis, but Mr. Zinbar's case was so far advanced that evidence of the disease had reached the peripheral blood circulation. He would probably be dead within the year.

Dr. Lugano arrived and was given the findings. He checked the slide with Dr. Bonner on the double-viewing microscope, and nodded as the pathologist pointed out the most incriminating signs in the smear. It was a terrible form of cancer the doctors were looking at. Near the end, the disease process eats away the bones of the spine and skull so that they are riddled with holes. Fractures are common and the patient feels a lot of back pain. They tire easily because of the anemia. And nosebleeds are common because the blood does not clot. Mr. Zinbar's disease was so far advanced it was strange that he had reported no symptoms.

□ □ □

Marc Micozzi had good reason to be nervous as he sat at the long table with eleven other students, waiting for Dr. John Kastor, the attending physician, to arrive.

Mark was about to perform one of the most intimidating rituals Medicine 200 students were required to do. It was a thing called "presenting to the attending."

The goal of these monologues, which can last up to half an hour, was for the junior person to verbally present the status of a new patient in sufficient detail for a senior physician to make an independent medical judgment.

The student had to get all the information himself from examining the patient and taking the medical history. In addition, the presentations were as stylized as a Japanese kabuki dance. Each nuance of the ceremony had to be mastered, with all the information being presented in a precise order that never varies.

Dr. Kastor rushed into the room and promptly took the seat at the head of the long table, which was the customary place for the attending. The resident told Dr. Kastor who would present the case, Dr. Kastor nodded to the student with a smile, and Marc slowly started the presentation.

He was in fine form. A large man of twenty-two with a neat mustache and the threat of a worried look on his face, Marc sat straight and tall at the table. His voice was deep and resonant and he picked up speed as he gained confidence, making his way through the intricacies of the presentation with practically no interruptions from the attending.

Never pausing or hesitating from insecurity, Marc's voice boomed out, taking his audience from chief complaint to patient profile to present illness to past medical history to family history to review of organ systems and functions to physical examination to laboratory studies to summary. And then, after more than twenty-five minutes, it was over, and Marc sat looking at Dr. Kastor, waiting for some sign.

At first, Dr. Kastor said nothing. He just continued to look at Marc. Then finally the attending spoke:

"Very nice presentation," Dr. Kastor said with a smile. "Very thorough and you thought it out well. It's one of the best presentations I've heard in this course."

Compliments like that were not passed out lightly, especially in the medical department of the HUP, the jewel in the crown of hospitals attended by Penn medical students, the medical Mecca, the hospital against which all other hospitals were measured and found lacking.

"But," Dr. Kastor continued before the compliment could be fully savored, "you took too long."

□ □ □

It takes a lot of intelligence and hard work to get through medical school, but it also helps to know how to play the game. Everyone played some form of the game—the students, interns, residents, and even the attendings, the full-fledged physicians with faculty appointments.

The goal of the game was never to look stupid and always to appear bright, even if it meant passing up an opportunity to learn something.

The students knew only too well that just about every doctor they came into formal contact with would fill out an evaluation form on them, so they were always on their toes.

Hence the more senior the doctor lecturing, the less frequently students would ask questions, for fear of looking stupid. The only exception to this was the clever question designed to demonstrate how much the student asking it knew.

One student was so adept at this tactic that he seldom asked a question that did not provoke some admiring comment from the instructor like, "That was a good question," or, "I'm glad you asked that." On an intern and resident level, a popular tactic was to quote generously from prestigious journals like the *New England Journal of Medicine* or *Lancet.*

When a student asked a question that stumped the intern, the standard ploy was for the intern to say: "I could explain that to you, but I think you'd get more out of it if you looked the answer up yourself."

Rarely did anyone say flat out that he did not know something. Rather, he gave an involved answer with several components in the hope that he might inadvertently hit upon the right one.

Amusingly, the only people who consistently would admit ignorance were the very senior men, the specialists, and they seemed to get some perverse pleasure out of saying, "I don't know," almost as though they were humble, simple people. This was a safe tactic, for at a place like the HUP, when the top specialist said he did not know, the assumption always was that only God knew.

Mr. Zinbar was watching *The Doctors* on the small television hanging in front of his face from an accordion support when Dr. Lugano arrived and introduced himself. Mr. Zinbar had the happy, buoyant, positive personality so common among salesmen and he looked Dr. Lugano straight in the eyes.

"No, I really feel great," Mr. Zinbar said. "Except for this stupid hand. I'm real active. Love my work. Love my children. Even love my wife." He laughed. Dr. Lugano didn't.

"Then there has been no change in your daily activities?" Dr. Lugano said.

"None at all," Mr. Zinbar said. "I tell you, I feel really great. Especially now, because me and the family are planning to go to Europe for the first time together. We expect it will be one of the best times of our lives."

Dr. Lugano almost winced, but he caught it. Dr. Lugano wasn't responding to Mr. Zinbar's joviality and the man was becoming aware of this.

"What about stairs?" Dr. Lugano asked.

"What do you mean 'what about stairs?' " Mr. Zinbar asked.

"Do you have any trouble going upstairs? I mean, do you stop to catch your breath or do you go up them much more slowly now?"

"Now that you mention it," Mr. Zinbar said, "I have been feeling tired lately. But I thought it was because I've been so busy, working and planning for the trip and all. I used to run up the stairs, but now I take them slowly, one at a time."

Dr. Lugano noted this on the clipboard resting on his lap.

The joviality was gone now. Mr. Zinbar was becoming suspicious. He wondered if this young doctor sitting in front of him knew something that he wasn't telling him.

"Do you ever get nosebleeds?" Dr. Lugano asked.

An unexpected explosion in a dark room couldn't have startled Mr. Zinbar more. Studying Dr. Lugano with a frightened stare, Mr. Zinbar said: "Yes. I've been getting nosebleeds every day recently."

□ □ □

Dr. Paul Mitnick, a young resident, waited until they were out of earshot of the patient before he asked the senior physician the question. The older doctor, a man in his late sixties or early seventies, was one of the most respected physicians in Philadelphia, though he had cut back his practice in recent years.

The patient in question would undoubtedly soon have a heart attack or some other potentially lethal complication, and Dr. Mitnick was seeking guidance. The older physician was the man's personal doctor and it was for him to make major decisions.

In effect Dr. Mitnick wanted to find out if they should try to save the man when the crisis comes.

In this modern era, it was possible to call a code in such cases, and doctors would come running in from all over the hospital, pound on the patient's chest, zap him with a jolt of electricity, and maybe bring him back to life.

Sometimes they might do this a half-dozen times on a single patient. With seriously ill, older patients, more often than not each resuscitation became more difficult as the process of repeated heart attacks slowly destroyed the heart or brain or other organs.

The older physician walked down the hall and sat down with Dr. Mitnick at the nurses' station. It had been a long day for him and he found these momentary rests refreshing. For a moment he pondered the question that Dr. Mitnick didn't ask outright and then talked a little philosophy instead of medicine.

"When my time comes, I don't think that cardiac arrest would be such a bad thing to happen. Would it serve any point to interfere? What can we offer him?"

He reviewed the medical situation and spoke about the cancer that had spread through the man's lungs and the kidneys that were just barely working and the man's senility. The older doctor nodded to the younger one and smiled.

"Yes," he said getting back up on his tired legs, "sometimes it is bad to do everything you can." Slowly he walked down the hall, leaving Dr. Mitnick at the nurses' station. He never really answered the implied question of whether a code should be called. But he didn't have to because he had made his answer clear.

It is difficult for new doctors to restrain themselves sometimes. They become so enmeshed in the technology and the increasingly varied options science is continually giving them that the patient is lost sight of.

In their endless conferences and case discussions, the medical men spend hours talking about a given patient's condition. They talk about increasing his blood pressure with this drug or stimulating his heart with that one.

They talk about x-ray studies that may answer a diagnostic question. Or they cite a report about a similar case published in a medical journal. They describe the intricacies of the disease process, drawing on incredibly sophisticated knowledge, but rarely do they ask the ultimate questions: Will the patient get better? Will he survive?

There seems to be a preoccupation with the next possible manipulation of drug or technique that will produce the next possible physiological effect, whether it be an increase in heart rate or a drop in blood pressure.

From such a process undoubtedly comes orderly, therapeutic progression. But the very detail also serves as an intellectual buffer from the enormity of what is involved.

This is so much the situation that after a lengthy case discussion, it almost comes as a surprise to walk into the patient's room and discover that all these lab reports, x-ray films, and medical charts represent a human being not very much different in form from the doctors who were talking about him.

The danger of overintellectualizing and hence dehumanizing medical care is a very real one, especially in a high-pressure academic institution like the HUP.

The faculty was forever reminding students to think in terms of patients, of total human beings, not disease processes. Referring to a patient as this gall bladder on the third floor or bad lungs on five invariably provoked a rebuke.

Dr. Kastor criticized the students whenever they used such words as male or female instead of man or woman. But so much of a medical student's training at this point centered on the basics of disease process and physiology that it was difficult not to think in terms of gall bladders and lungs rather than people.

Patients were much more people and medicine was much less perfect in the eyes of the older physicians, trained in an era when medicine couldn't do so much and made humble by years of trying to treat diseases that science was not yet capable of treating.

□ □ □

It was the hematologist who finally told Mr. Zinbar what the situation was. She told him how he had a form of blood cancer. She told him that it was serious. But, she said, there were some drugs that they could give that would help for a while.

She told him that he would have to come to the hospital frequently. And that the drugs were very powerful but very imperfect so there would be a lot of bad reactions. She didn't tell him that he probably wouldn't live another year.

Mr. Zinbar listened, but the implications of what was being said were too much for him to handle immediately.

"Will the drugs cure the disease?" he asked.

The hematologist shook her head. "We don't have any drugs that can cure this disease. The best we can do is control it for a while."

"If you can control it does that mean after a while I'll get over it?" he asked. Again the hematologist shook her head.

"Oh," Mr. Zinbar said. He thought silently for a while. Then he asked, "But the drugs can control the disease?"

"For a while," the hematologist said.

Mr. Zinbar shrugged his shoulders. He still didn't realize what was being told to him.

"It's funny," he said after thinking for a moment. "I couldn't see any reason for getting so worked up over this little cut of mine."

22

He was an ancient white-haired man of eighty-six with arms no thicker than his thin wrists. He lay in a bed in Pennsylvania Hospital. And though dressed only in a scanty hospital gown, and weakened by illness, the man had dignity.

He did not object to the poking and probing that was part of the physical examination given to him by medical student Howard Levy, a youth almost one quarter the old man's age.

And he answered every question put to him by Howard with perception and sometimes wit. But something was bothering the old man. He waited until Howard was through and then told him about it:

"I will answer all the questions you ask," the man said. "And you can do all the tests you want. But under no circumstances will I submit to surgery."

The old man's skin and the whites of his eyes were an obvious yellow. He was not in pain, though. Oddly, the lack of pain was an ominous sign. Even a second-year student knew what painless jaundice usually meant in someone of this great age.

Billirubin, a red pigment from the bile made in the liver and stored in the gall bladder, was building up in the blood and turning the man's skin yellow. Something obviously was blocking the bile ducts from the gall bladder and liver. But because there was no pain, gallstones were not the problem. Most likely the obstruction was caused by a tumor. Uncorrected, such an obstruction is lethal. The only treatment: surgery.

□ □ □

Pennsylvania Hospital was on the edge of Society Hill, an affluent, reconstructed Colonial area in Philadelphia. It was one of the seven hospitals that Penn medical students went to for training. It was unlike any other hospital they would ever serve in.

Part hospital, part museum, Pennsylvania Hospital was a friendly place for medical students. The standards were higher than in most community hospitals, but the pressures were small.

Scholarly one-upmanship was less often seen there than at the HUP. The pace was slower. Some of the students felt it was less exciting and demanding, while others welcomed the more relaxed rapport among interns and residents.

It was hard for anyone to forget that Pennsylvania Hospital was the nation's first, founded in 1751, by, of course, Benjamin Franklin. The students were reminded of this whenever they walked by Benjamin West's *Christ Healing the Sick* in the lobby, or the 1,100 brass plaques honoring every intern who had worked in Pennsylvania Hospital since Jacob Ehrenzeller did so in 1773, or the century-old wisteria bushes in the beautiful gardens outside.

Housing the oldest surgical amphitheater in the United States, Pennsylvania Hospital was also a museum, and administrator H. Robert Cathcart treated it with the veneration a museum deserved. The hospital was impeccably clean with gleaming, polished marble floors and brass shined to a sparkle.

Vacuum cleaners were forever roaring up and down the carpeted hallways, making it difficult for the doctors in their whispered bedside conferences to hear one another. Cathcart's mania for cleanliness had even put a huge powered vacuum cleaner to work on the sidewalks outside the historic walls of his beloved hospital.

□ □ □

Standing outside the old man's room on morning rounds, Howard presented the case to the attending, Dr. D. Jeffery Hartzell, a small mild-mannered physician who always seemed preoccupied with secret, gentle thoughts. A sandwich wrapped in a clear plastic wrap poked out of the pocket of his white hospital coat and he wore a pin that read: "I'm Proud to Work at the Nation's First Hospital."

Howard said he thought he felt a mass in the man's abdomen. He said the man had been vomiting after eating. He told about the billirubin count being high, and the man losing a lot of weight in the past few months.

Finally, after Howard was finished, Dr. Hartzell asked him what he thought the trouble was.

"I think he probably has a GI tumor with metastasis to the liver," Howard said without hesitation. Dr. Hartzell agreed.

"CRT in the CCU," the voice on the overhead loudspeaker said without emotion. "CRT in the CCU." This was an emergency call for the coronary resuscitation team. Someone's heart had stopped beating in the coronary-care unit and doctors and nurses were needed immediately to try to save him.

The house staff clustered around Dr. Hartzell ignored the call, though, because the CCU was in another building and other members of the resuscitation team would respond. The team of doctors and students went into the old man's room and Dr. Hartzell was introduced.

The old man was lying in bed, staring at the shadows made by the sunlight streaming through his window, when the group of doctors and students filed into the room. Dr. Hartzell asked the patient for permission to examine him. The old man nodded.

Gently, Dr. Hartzell lifted up the hospital gown and felt the man's belly, seeking the outline of his liver. The vomiting had become worse since the man had arrived in the hospital because the obstruction was becoming more severe.

After Dr. Hartzell was finished, he motioned to the two other students in the group, and they felt for the liver. A few questions were asked and the interview was ended.

"Thank you for talking to us," Dr. Hartzell said, squeezing the old man's hand. The group filed out of the room to the hallway, where the conference resumed.

"What do you think, Warren?" Dr. Hartzell asked, addressing first-year resident Dr. Warren Kurnick. "What are the top candidates on your list?"

"Tumor, tumor, tumor," Dr. Kurnick said. "Everything else would be low on my list."

A few yards down the hall, Mr. Taylor, a sixty-seven-year-old stroke patient, was making a commotion again, and the nurses, exasperated by his constant yelling and bullying, were yelling back at him to behave.

He had been only partly disabled by the stroke and did not need to be in the hospital. But all nursing homes contacted had refused to take him because the welfare payments for his care were too low. So for 159 days he had occupied a $181-a-day hospital room, watching color television and yelling at nurses.

Dr. Hartzell ignored the yelling and the approaching roar of a vacuum cleaner coming down the hall, concentrating on the discussion about the old man.

Someone asked: Why do surgery if tests showed that the man's body was filled with inoperable cancer. Why subject a man of this age to the pain and inconvenience of surgery if the outlook is hopeless anyhow?

Dr. Hartzell nodded in response to the questions, indicating that he understood why they were being asked.

Yes, it was true that the outlook for the man was grim. But there are different ways to die, the more knowledgeable in the group said, each contributing a bit to the discussion. The biliary obstruction would probably kill in a matter of weeks and the death could be very painful.

If the surgeons relieved the obstruction and removed whatever cancer they could reach, the old man might be given a few more months. More important, he probably would die the peaceful death of uremic poisoning. Wastes would build up in his blood, he would drift in and out of consciousness and then finally slip off into death.

There was always the chance—admittedly a very remote chance—that the surgeons would go in and find something other than a cancer causing the problem, something that could be cured.

But first there would have to be surgery. They would wait for the test results to come in so they could provide the old man with specific information when they talked to him. Until then nothing would be said.

□ □ □

Usually after morning rounds, doctors and students in the Spruce Street building would have breakfast in Ben's Den, a luncheonette on the first floor. Frequently business would be transacted over coffee and danish, but there would be a lot of nonmedical talk too.

Howard was a self-assured, twenty-three-year-old graduate of Haverford College, where he had studied chemistry. Unlike many of his classmates, Howard had adopted a somewhat humorous attitude toward medicine's deficiencies.

He was critical of the many doctors who he felt had enormous egos and who wrongly accepted the role of God thrust on them by their patients. Too much of medicine was dogmatic, he thought, and he expressed these feelings openly.

Howard could not have been assigned to a more suitable intern than the twenty-five-year-old Dr. Kurnick.

Dr. Kurnick was no egotistic, dogmatic physician. Instead, he was constantly counteracting the ponderous posturing of his more serious peers with wit and satire.

Sitting around the coffee containers and buns, he would poke fun at the humorless ways of some of his peers and then amusingly chastise a student who said she had a "gut feeling" about a diagnosis.

"Students are not allowed to have gut feelings," he said with exaggerated disapproval. "Students are supposed to read and find the answers in books. Only fifty-year-old physicians are entitled to gut feelings."

The growing group of people around the small table in Ben's Den was joined by Dr. Jane Churco, an intern assigned to the coronary care unit, and her surgeon husband, Alan.

"How'd you make out with that code?" Dr. Kurnick asked, referring to the cardiac resuscitation team call sounded over the loudspeaker earlier in the morning.

"No, we lost him," she said, buttering a bagel. They talked briefly about the surgery and the subsequent shock that led to the patient's death.

Then the conversation turned to happier topics. They joked about how Pennsylvania Hospital had more vacuum cleaners than any other hospital in the city, but only two operable electrocardiographs.

And how dental students have more outgoing personalities, more time, more parties, and more girl friends than medical students.

□ □ □

The sixty-seven-year-old man looked awful. Four bottles hung over his head, dripping fluids and nutrients into his veins. A blue plastic tube attached to a ventilator pressured oxygen into his ailing lungs.

Food was forced into his stomach through a nasogastric tube taped to his nose. And the fluid wastes from his body were collected in a plastic bag hung from his bed. Potent antibiotics needed to fight his pneumonia had already made him deaf, and his right eye was opaque from a cataract. He was only half-conscious.

He formed words with a toothless mouth, and seemed to be saying to intern Thomas Ziobrowski, "I'm dying." Someone thought he was saying that he wanted to die.

Weakened by an undiagnosed thyroid condition, Mr. Droke had come to the emergency room with advanced pneumonia. Now the intensive-care nurses were working at his bedside around the clock to keep him alive.

What was remarkable about this case was that if they could pull him through the pneumonia, it would be easy to control his thyroid condition with available drugs. Despite his pitiful condition, the man might be saved.

Across the small intensive care in a corner bed was another patient, a much younger man, only twenty-eight, who would never leave the unit. He had an extremely unusual genetic defect that claimed its victims in the late twenties or thirties, after they had fathered children and passed the trait on to those children.

It was a progressive neurologic disease that eventually left the stricken with virtually no voluntary movements at all.

This was the stage this man had reached. He could not raise his head or move his arms or even talk. He communicated by moving his eyelids to indicate "yes" or "no," a feat he could just barely accomplish.

Nearby at the nurses' station in the ICU, Drs. Kurnick and Ziobrowski were talking about Mr. Droke's condition in particular and the problems of medicine in general.

Howard said he was becoming more firmly resolved in his decision to go into emergency medicine, though he still had not made up his mind definitely.

As they talked they could hear a nurse slapping the chest of the neurologic patient, trying to clear the congestion from his lungs.

□ □ □

Howard presented the case of the old man with the gall bladder obstruction to the incredible Dr. Louis R. Dinon, who ran the student training program at Pennsylvania Hospital with the same exaggerated breathless enthusiasm that a teacher might use to generate interest in a grammar school class.

He tended to belabor the obvious, wear bow ties and short cropped hair, and liked to pretend that he was tough. He was not the cool sophisticated university hospital physician—in fact he was even a little corny—but the students all liked the fifty-year-old Dr. Dinon because he cared about them. He was enthusiastic about teaching and spent a couple of hours a week with each student listening to case presentations.

"Jaundice and dark urine," Dr. Dinon said, excitedly whispering the words Howard had just used in presenting the old man's case. "Jaundice and dark urine means hepatic involvement. Wonderful. Wonderful. Go on."

Dr. Dinon sat behind the desk in his small office and Howard sat in a school chair with an arm for taking notes. Howard continued, finally coming to the lab figures.

"A billirubin of twenty-five!" Dr. Dinon yelled with such excited enthusiasm that it startled Howard, who smiled awkwardly. "Yes. That is very high. But we already knew it was obstructive disease, didn't we? The dark urine." He whispered the words.

For two and a half hours Dr. Dinon worked over the case as Howard became increasingly concerned about the time. It was getting late and Howard's brother had tickets for the Flyer's hockey playoffs that night.

Dr. Dinon agreed that more tests could be done, but it was already clear to him. The old man needed surgery.

Howard nodded, thanked Dr. Dinon, and rushed off to call his brother.

□ □ □

The old man's condition had become markedly worse and he could just barely sit up in the chair near the window where he liked to read in the sun.

The vomiting had become more frequent because of the obstruction, and now the man had a tube threaded through his nose and into his stomach to relieve the problem.

Even with this, he managed to maintain his proud bearing, sitting in the sun with the newspaper folded on his lap. But the repeated tests and the growing institutional dependence were beginning to weaken his will against further medical measures. He still did not want surgery, but he was less emphatic.

Over the coming days the test results began to come in, and intern Jerry Gabry began to amass the data he would need to discuss the case with the man's private physician and possibly the old man himself.

A radiologic scan of the liver showed the ducts to be dilated, indicating obstruction, but no tumor mass was seen.

The chest x-rays were negative. Another film showing the small bowel outlined by the radiologic opaque barium was also negative. The man's liver was large, but there were no holes indicating a cancerous process.

Though all the tests continued to be negative, the doctors clung to their tentative diagnosis that a tumor was obstructing the bile ducts.

Finally, an upper gastrointestinal test showed a mass in the duodenum, the beginning of the small intestine, where bile from the gall bladder and liver enters to participate in the digestion process.

This was the cause of the problem. The diagnosis had been confirmed.

Specialists from gastroenterology and surgery would be called in to review the findings, examine the old man, and make final plans.

Howard was particularly involved in this case because it was very interesting from an educational standpoint. The problem was a common one and many tests had to be done to verify a disease with almost classic symptoms.

There was a sense of drama as the diagnostic pieces fell into place and the confirmation was achieved. The delicate business of the man's refusing surgery everyone agreed he should have heightened the tension surrounding the case. But despite Howard's involvement and the dramatic buildup, he never found out if the man finally broke down and agreed to surgery and if he did what the outcome was.

This was Howard's last week on the Medicine 200 rotation and the matter hadn't been resolved by the time he left the rotation Friday evening. Monday would be a different rotation in a different hospital with different house staff officers and different patients. That was one of the more irksome things about medical education. The students were forever moving on, and involvement and commitment was something that wasn't easy to maintain. Howard had intended to call back to find out, but he was rushed on the other rotation and never did find the time.

Once again the warm weather had returned and the second year of medical school was ending. It didn't seem like it was over because there was no academic structure to separate the second from the third year or the third from the fourth. And the hospital rotations went straight through the year with no regard for the months or school terms or other extraneous considerations.

23

It was a hot night in June, and the only person walking along the dark sidewalk in the west Philadelphia ghetto was a sixteen-year-old boy coming home from a basketball game. Suddenly a shot rang out and the boy fell to the ground near death with a bullet in his head.

Police responded immediately and took him to nearby Presbyterian Hospital, where the boy died. The ghetto tragedy was a senseless murder for reasons the police would never be able to determine. But some momentary good came from it because instead of sending the body to the morgue the physicians hooked the boy up to a respirator and kept the heart beating. Being young and, until the moment of the shooting, in perfect health, the youth had strong healthy kidneys that could be transplanted into people with end-stage kidney disease.

The Presbyterian Hospital doctors immediately called the Delaware Valley Transplant Program, a coordinating agency that collected kidneys from area hospitals and then distributed them to surgeons who had patients needing kidneys. A representative of the program contacted the boy's parents, explained the need for such organs, and obtained permission for them to be removed and given to other patients. One of the boy's kidneys went to St. Christopher's Hospital for Children and the other went to the HUP.

□ □ □

It was early in the morning, but Ron was already in the bed in the dialysis unit at the HUP. Clear plastic tubes, red with Ron's blood, led from his arm to the dialysis machine next to the bed.

Ron had been coming to the unit three times a week for the past eight months. Each time he came he wondered if it would be the last time. Always there was the hope that today would be the day that they'd find the kidney for him. He didn't like the prospect of surgery, but it was far preferable to being held prisoner by the machine.

He had waited so long that he was getting angry at the doctors and the medical system and the disease that had done this to him. Everything he wanted depended on getting the kidney. And going to the unit three times a week was depressing because he could see his future there in the form of more seriously ill patients. These were the men and women who had been on the machine for years, and their bodies were losing the fight.

Every now and then Ron would come into the unit and find out that one of his dialysis-unit friends was no longer alive. And Ron and the other people in the unit would wonder then when their time would come. It was almost like being on death row and watching the prison guards take fellow cellmates off to the electric chair, wondering when they'd be standing at your door.

It was 8:30 when Dr. Grossman came over to Ron and smiled. Without any other emotion he said that they had obtained a kidney. The match appeared good. He asked him if he was willing to undergo surgery now. If the answer was yes they'd have to start preparing him immediately because the operation would be done at 5:00 that night.

Kidneys are very fragile, and even with the best preservation methods they can't be kept viable for more than a day or so at best. Ron had no doubts. He wanted the kidney. Dr. Grossman nodded and left.

The surgeon would be Dr. Clyde F. Barker, the principal transplant surgeon at the HUP. The kidney had already arrived from Presbyterian Hospital in an organ-preservation thermos that didn't look much different from a picnic cooler.

Rikki was contacted at home and by five o'clock was already in the green scrub suit of the operating room, walking beside Ron's litter as they wheeled him down the hall to surgery. She and Ron had discussed it many times before and agreed that she should be with him during the operation, perhaps even assisting.

Rikki had developed a theory that the medical system wrongly created a patient/doctor dichotomy in which the patient was left helpless, no longer in control of his fate. Relinquishing any say in what was done to him, the patient ended up losing his dignity, independence, and, to some extent, sense of worth. This was true, she felt, not only for the patients but for their relatives as well. She thought it was important that they all participate in the medical process so that they could grow with the medical crisis rather than be divided and made helpless by it. This is why she wanted to be with Ron in the operating room.

Her strongly felt opinions on this matter were shared by many of her liberal classmates and even several doctors. But they were not shared by Dr. Clyde F. Barker, who just shook his head when he saw her walk into the operating room with Ron, dressed in the greens with a mask around her neck.

No, she would have to leave. He said he didn't think it was fair to her or the people caring for Ron in the operating room. Her presence, he said, would put undue strain on the doctors and nurses. And should something go wrong, it would be devastating for all concerned.

Rikki wasn't happy about it, but she left, pushing through the swinging doors of the O.R., as she felt a sense of helplessness flood over her.

The operation went well, and soon they were wheeling Ron back to his room. The kidney was in fine condition. It made urine right away, indicating that it was functioning well in Ron's body, and for the moment everything looked fine.

The first couple of postoperative days went well also. The surgical wound was healing as it should. Ron continued to urinate. And the young couple began to envision a future distinct and separate from the machine. They started thinking of going on musical tours and of doing a lot of other things that involved travel, daydreams that were not possible before.

Ron started hiccuping on the third day after the operation. It seemed like a silly annoyance after all he had gone through. But to the doctors, this was an ominous sign. It meant that the uremia had come back. The toxins building up in Ron's blood were causing neuromuscular irritability, which resulted in the hiccuping. Ron's temperature started climbing and soon it was 103 degrees. And his blood pressure went up. The crisis they had all been dreading had begun—immunologic rejection.

Ron's body had started to kill the transplant organ. It was a massive rejection episode, one of the worst Dr. Grossman had ever seen. Four times they dialyzed Ron to give the new kidney assistance. Drugs were pumped into him to counteract the immunologic response. But nothing would work.

Ron was in agony. Everytime he hiccuped he stretched the wound site of the surgery and sharp pains would cut into his side. They gave him pain-killing drugs, but they didn't help much. Rikki sneaked some pot into the hospital and Ron smoked it on the sly in the bathroom. Surprisingly it relaxed him and helped the pain more than the morphine and Thorazine the nurses had been giving him.

On the eighth day Dr. Barker came into Ron's room and told him the bad news. They would have to remove the transplanted kidney. It had been destroyed by the rejection process. Ron would have to go back on the machine again.

24

The doctors and nurses knew that the man in 1602 was a high-risk patient and might not survive the upcoming operation.

Bedridden and made a virtual cripple by a heart that had been severely weakened by repeated attacks, the man had come to the HUP hoping that surgeons could make him strong again.

Open-heart surgery had become reasonably safe in recent years, but two big problems made this man's surgery more risky than most. His heart had been weakened by five attacks and might not withstand the stress of the operation.

And the man was a Jehovah's Witness. His religious convictions would not allow him to receive blood transfusions. If he should require blood, which was a distinct possibility, the surgeons would have to stand by and let him die.

Lying in his bed, with a Bible and a copy of the Witnesses' periodical, *Watchtower,* on the nightstand next to him, George Hinden looked deceptively strong. He was a fat man with a tight, nervous smile and thick glasses. He never mentioned his fears, but they showed in his face and in the vociferous way he answered the questions Matt Lotysh asked him for the preoperative medical history.

Dressed in the wrinkled green scrub suit of the surgeon, Matt sat on a chair close to Mr. Hinden's bed with a medical chart on his lap. As a third-year medical student assigned to the cardiothoracic surgery service, Matt was responsible for examining and interviewing patients admitted to the service.

In the five weeks he had been doing this, Matt had assisted surgeons in dozens of operations similar to the one Mr. Hinden would have, and blood transfusions usually weren't needed. Usually, but not always.

"The Heavenly Father lays down the law," Mr. Hinden said nervously, trying to explain why he couldn't accept blood transfusions—a point that Matt deliberately had not raised.

"It says in Acts fifteen twenty-nine that you must abstain from meats offered to idols and from blood and things strangled and from fornication. . . ."

Matt nodded; he would not challenge Mr. Hinden's interpretation of the Scriptures, written thousands of years before there was such a thing as a blood transfusion. This was not for Matt to do. Many physicians had discussed this matter with Mr. Hinden long before he was admitted to the hospital. The patient was well aware of the added risks and had made his decision. It was Matt's responsibility to help prepare him for surgery and provide whatever reassurance he could.

Would it be permissible, Matt asked gently, to take blood from him, store it in a bottle and return his own blood to him later should an emergency develop during surgery? Mr. Hinden shook his head.

"It's all right for my blood to leave my body and go through the heart machine," Mr. Hinden said, indicating an unusual sophistication about such procedures, "as long as it always remains a part of my circulation. That wouldn't be so if you stored it in a bottle, even for a few hours."

Matt nodded, assuring him that all the medical personnel who would deal with him were aware of his religious beliefs. They would respect them —no matter what happened.

□ □ □

Having started their third year of medical school, the students in the class of '78 were now midway through their medical education.

The main difference between a third-year student and a second-year student was that in a few advanced courses the third-year student had some responsibility and was depended upon by other members of the hospital's medical team. He was not there merely for educational purposes.

Though his work was closely supervised and frequently done over by members of the house staff, the third-year student was responsible for admitting new patients to the floors, performing routine care and gathering information for the preparation of the medical charts that nurses and physicians used in caring for each patient.

The students in the class of '78 had come a long way both professionally and personally since the muggy September morning in 1974 when they gathered for the first time to begin their medical careers.

* Mark Reber was more convinced than ever that he wanted to go into pediatrics. Using the liberal elective program at Penn, he already had taken neonatal studies at the HUP, general pediatrics and pediatric surgery at Children's Hospital, and infectious diseases at Columbia University Children's Hospital in New York. Earlier in the year he had married a social worker from New York.

* Andrew Henderson's wife, Valerie, a third-year medical student at Thomas Jefferson University, had just given birth to a daughter, Heather Marie. Valerie had kept up with her studies right up to delivery, and now a neighbor would take care of the child while the two continued their education.

Andrew had all but made up his mind to specialize in pediatrics. His intention was to open a group practice in South Philadelphia with his wife, who was interested in obstetrics-gynecology, and other black physicians.

When Andrew was a child in the Southward project of south Philadelphia, the only doctor in his neighborhood was a white physician who, after being shot once in his office, accepted only patients he knew.

Things had improved somewhat but many such neighborhoods still lacked physicians, and Andrew wanted to fill that need.

He was somewhat saddened that some of his fellow black students at Penn were thinking of going into specialties like pathology or radiology, fields that attracted many white students but that seemed far removed from the needs of black communities.

* Walter Tsou, the eager twenty-three-year-old who began medical school with so much nervous energy, had grown a little weary of its constant demands. He had been working constantly since the very start, having spent the first summer vacation on a surgery rotation and the second one in a medical program in Appalachia.

Though he admitted that he was beginning to feel weighed down, he didn't intend to relax until next summer. The third year was particularly important to medical students because that was the year the professors look at when writing letters of recommendation for hospital internships.

The right internship can make a big difference in a physician's career, and after all his work Walter had no intention of taking any chances.

Not all students were so concerned with such tactics. In fact, many were using this term as a midpoint break, or as a chance to get away from the Penn campus.

* Steve Levine was taking a rotation in gastroenterology at the University of California in San Francisco.

* Marc Micozzi was on a year-long scholarship out of the country studying tropical medicine in Manila.

□ □ □

After he finished examining Mr. Hinden and reviewing the medical data provided by physicians and a variety of sophisticated tests, Matt realized that this was a very sick patient.

The three principal arteries feeding Mr. Hinden's heart had been seriously clogged by the plaque of atherosclerosis, which, like caked rust in old pipes, had cut the flow of blood to a trickle. This accounted for the many heart attacks.

The repeated attacks had scarred the heart, and the left ventricle, the main pumping chamber, had lost much of its ability to contract and thus pump blood. This was particularly menacing because Mr. Hinden's heart needed all possible reserve to endure the extra demands that surgery would place on it.

The heart surgeon, Dr. MacVaugh, planned to take extra veins from Mr. Hinden's leg and patch them around the clogged places in the coronary arteries, like setting up a detour around an obstacle in a road.

Developed only five years earlier, this procedure, called a coronary artery bypass graft, had become one of the most frequently performed operations in the country. It provided dramatic relief of symptoms—patients who were barely able to sit up before surgery were walking around the hospital days after the operation—but there was still no conclusive proof that it extended the life expectancy of heart patients.

Dr. MacVaugh would put Mr. Hinden on a heart-lung machine, a device that would keep the blood circulating through Mr. Hinden's body while the surgeon stopped his heart to make repairs. The blood would leave Mr. Hinden's body through a tube coming from an artery on one side of his heart; enter the machine, where it would be loaded with oxygen and drained of carbon dioxide; and then be pumped back into him through a vein on the other side of his heart.

After the repairs to Mr. Hinden's heart were completed, the blood would be routed through the heart again, the organ would be electrically shocked back to beating, and then Mr. Hinden would be taken off the machine.

Sometimes, however, surgeons would run into trouble when they took the patient off the pump. The heart refused to start beating again. The blood pressure would drop. And the patient would have to go back on the machine while the doctors attempted to correct the problem with drugs, fluids, and blood transfusions.

It was in those final stages, when normal functions were to be restored, that the doctors feared they would have the biggest problems with Mr. Hinden's heart.

Mr. Hinden was scheduled for surgery at 11:00 the next morning. This was late in the day to start such a procedure, but Dr. MacVaugh had three other major operations that morning. His first patient, who would get a heart valve, was scheduled for 6:00 A.M.

While Matt was making note of the drugs and other procedures Mr. Hinden would require before his operation, a second-year medical student came up to him inquiring about the possibility of interviewing and examining a patient.

With impressive command of the situation, Matt told him the best patient to check, explained what type of information to get, how to get specimens for lab studies, and what to include in the medical history. In obvious deference to Matt's position as a third-year student, the second-year student set out to do what he was told.

Matt finished Mr. Hinden's medical record, noted on the jacket cover that it should be checked by the nursing staff for implementation, and put it back with the other charts. The final process had been completed in the series of events leading to Mr. Hinden's operation.

□ □ □

Cardiovascular surgery has come to represent, in the public mind at least, the great achievement of modern medicine. When people talk about medical advances, open-heart surgery and heart transplantation are invariably mentioned. Many doctors believe that these things are probably overrated, just as the achievements of cancer therapy are underrated.

While Matt was busy on the sixth floor participating in these miracles of modern science, fellow third-year student Travis Tolly was working on the third floor in the oncology unit, where thirty-three-year-old Dr. John Glick was trying to overcome the pessimism of both patients and physicians toward the treatment of cancer.

Cancer therapy had lacked a breakthrough with dramatic public appeal like heart transplantations. It remained a sad fact that cancer was largely incurable and, with the exception of skin cancer and a few very rare cancers like some forms of leukemia and Hodgkin's disease, the advances had been measured in terms of years of extra life rather than cures.

But those extra years were important, and the advent of multidrug therapy, to join the old standbys of surgery and radiation, constituted a breakthrough equal to that of cardiovascular surgery. If nothing else, this was the message that the energetic, almost evangelistic, Dr. Glick was trying to deliver to Travis Tolly and anyone else who would listen.

Walking through the hospital, past the beds of one cancer patient after another, Dr. Glick emitted an optimism that made cancer seem much less ominous—though almost all of the inpatients he talked to were in the final stages of a disease that would claim them in a few months or, at most, a year or two.

It was a sad business, despite Dr. Glick's optimism, that twenty-three-year-old Travis was exposed to.

There was a lovely woman, with a gentle smile and sensitive eyes, who was trying to keep the devastation of her disease from her husband. They were sending her home with a drug that would make her feel better. The drug would work only for a month or so, and then the woman's body would become resistant to it. But that didn't matter now because her liver had been destroyed by the disease and she probably wouldn't live much longer than a month anyway.

The drugs for cancer chemotherapy were used in such complex regimens and combinations that it now took highly specialized medical teams to employ them effectively.

At Penn, for instance, most of the cancer drugs were administered by four specially trained nurses who spent all their time in the cancer clinic or going from floor to floor implementing the oncologists' orders. The floor nurses usually were not permitted to give the drugs themselves.

As recently as five years earlier, medical students at Penn had no unified courses or clinical rotations in cancer. Instead they had to learn about the disease in bits and pieces as they rotated through different services such as medicine, surgery, gynecology. Now they had a four-week clinical rotation in cancer, in which they dealt with patients, as well as an eight-week didactic course.

Interestingly, much of the time Dr. Glick spent with the students was devoted to dealing with nonmedical problems, the kind of things that physicians in the past consistently ignored because of their own fears and feelings of inadequacy when confronting cancer.

What Dr. Glick emphasized was providing psychological support to terrified patients.

On other services, attending physicians usually spent only a minute or two at the bedside of each patient and then quickly moved on, discussing the case with their entourage. But Dr. Glick spent a lot of time with each patient, especially the new ones who had just been admitted and had not accepted the fact of their cancer. Typical of this was a woman who had just been admitted with a blood cancer.

Petrified with fear, she sat up in bed as Dr. Glick introduced himself. Her tension was obvious.

"Do you know what's wrong with you?" Dr. Glick asked, sitting down close to her.

"Yes," she said, appealing to him with her eyes. "I have cancer."

"And what does that mean to you?" he continued.

"It means I'm going to die," she said.

For the next fifteen minutes, Dr. Glick talked about cancer and the myths that surrounded it, about all the drugs that were available now, and about the aggressive way they were going to attack the disease in her body.

The woman was still obviously scared when Dr. Glick and his team left, but she thanked him repeatedly and seemed a little less alone than she had appeared before he sat down to talk to her.

□ □ □

Mr. Hinden was calm on the morning of the heart operation. He had been slightly sedated with tranquilizers, but he was alert and talked easily with his visitors. He had already sent his Bible and other possessions home. After surgery they would take him to the intensive-care unit, where there was no room for such things.

It was a gray rainy day, and rivulets of rain, blown by a cold wind, danced across the window as Mr. Hinden talked about his plans. When he recovered from the operation, he said, he was going to take a trip to Europe with his family. He had always wanted to do that, but couldn't because of the heart disease, which had curtailed such activities for the past ten years.

Mr. Hinden realized that he had no guarantee that the surgery would be successful, but he was ready for whatever happened. He started talking about the Kingdom on Earth and the new system God would create as described in Revelation.

"God will wipe away the tears from everyone's eyes," he said. "It will be wonderful and there will be no more sorrow or crying or pain. And there will be no more death."

It was clear now why Mr. Hinden had been so adamant about not permitting transfusions. No matter what the doctors said about the problems and dangers, who would want to trade a place in such a kingdom as he envisioned for a few pints of blood?

A few minutes later Mr. Hinden's reverie was broken when a nurse came in with a tray of syringes. It was time to get ready for the operation.

Downstairs on the fourth floor, the open-heart surgical teams were already busy with earlier operations.

Dr. MacVaugh was in Operating Room One, surrounded by green-robed personnel and equipment, finishing a heart-valve operation. In Operating Room Two, Matt and other members of the second team talked across the unconscious and exposed form of Dr. MacVaugh's second patient, waiting for the surgeon to get through with the first operation.

Already anesthetized, the patient was ready for the vein graft. Dr. MacVaugh's assistant had cut through his breast bone, exposing the heart, and the veins that would be used had already been taken from his leg.

It took more than two hours to get a patient ready for such operations on the heart, and the various phases of the surgery had to be timed with precision so that Dr. MacVaugh could move from operating room to operating room without waiting.

The surgery on the heart itself was the most difficult part of the operation and this was the only part Dr. MacVaugh usually did. The less difficult aspects of the procedure were done by other surgeons, who exposed the heart and then closed up the patient after Dr. MacVaugh was finished.

The mortality rate in open-heart surgery was inversely proportional to the number of operations a surgeon did. The more procedures he performed each week, the lower his mortality rate. Dr. MacVaugh's rate of about 6 percent was among the lowest in the country.

The first three operations took two hours longer than planned. It wasn't until 2:30 that Dr. MacVaugh started implanting three grafts into Mr. Hinden's heart.

Dr. MacVaugh was surprised by the extent of scarring he saw. Each of Mr. Hinden's five heart attacks had left behind slashes of tough white scar tissue that curtailed the heart's ability to pump blood. Nevertheless, the first phase of the operation went without incident.

At no time did the blood pressure drop significantly. The heart-lung machine kept the blood amply perfused with oxygen. And, amazingly, Mr. Hinden lost only a few ounces of blood.

It wasn't until Dr. MacVaugh ordered Mr. Hinden off the machine that trouble began.

The technician turned the machine off, routing Mr. Hinden's blood through his heart again. And then they shocked his heart to start it up. But instead of responding to the electric shocks with a nice steady beat, the heart pulsed crazily, swelling larger with each beat. His heart was fibrillating. It was beating wildly in an ineffective way. No blood was being circulated.

"Let's go back on bypass," Dr. MacVaugh said calmly.

Dr. MacVaugh and his assistant, Dr. Donald Tomasello, stood on either side of the operating table, staring down at the exposed, sick heart.

Frequently under such circumstances the heart will repair itself if it is given a few minutes of rest while the heart-lung machine does the pumping. After a few minutes the machine was shut off again, but again the heart failed to respond.

"Back on bypass," said one of the green-robed surgeons.

"Pressure fifty," the anesthesiologist called out. The blood pressure was dangerously low. "It's beginning to rise now."

"Better get the balloon," another voice said. The circulating nurse responded quickly, *click-clacking* out of the operating room on the wooden clogs she wore. She almost ran out. It was the only sign in the otherwise calm operating room that anything was wrong.

Mr. Hinden's ailing heart would be aided by a balloon that would be threaded into the aorta, the heart's major artery.

Alternately filling and emptying with helium from a hose attached to a portable machine in the operating room, the balloon would act like a pump, helping the heart to push blood through the circulatory system. All three units—the balloon, the heart-lung machine and the heart itself—are, after all, pumps. But unlike the heart-lung machine, which damages blood and can be used only for a few hours, the balloon can partially assist the heart for days, supporting the patient in the intensive-care unit.

Mr. Hinden's blood pressure improved. Again he was taken off the machine. But his heart would not pump properly, and once more the pressure dropped. This was extremely dangerous. The circulating blood cannot perfuse the brain and other vital organs with adequate amounts of oxygen if its pressure drops too low.

To anticipate this danger, the anesthesiologist took frequent blood samples during the operation, sending them to the laboratory to learn how much oxygen was being absorbed by the blood.

"What can you give us?" a voice called out to the heart-lung machine technician. The surgeons wanted more pressure. "We need everything you've got."

"We've given you everything."

Again the staccato of the *click-clacking* shoes. The nurse pushed through the operating room's swinging doors with the machine that would inflate the balloon.

"Better go back on the machine."

Mr. Hinden already had been prepared to receive the balloon. It was quickly threaded through a blood vessel to the aorta. One of the anesthesiologists started working the machine.

"Get the paddles ready."

They were about to hit Mr. Hinden's heart again with a jolt from the electric paddles. Everyone stood back to avoid getting shocked.

"Hit it!"

The body jerked, but the heart didn't respond.

"Turn the balloon on."

It didn't help.

"Turn the balloon off."

"He's fibrillating."

"Stand clear . . . hit it!"

Once again the electric shock.

The operating-room phone buzzed. It was the laboratory. The gasses in Mr. Hinden's blood were bad. Not enough oxygen. Too much carbon dioxide. The acid balance was off.

"Give him a shot of lidocaine."

The anesthesiologists responded to the crisis. Drugs were given to force the blood pressure up and strengthen the heart. Sodium bicarbonate was injected into the lines to improve the blood gas picture.

The pressure on the heart-lung machine could not be maintained. There was not enough blood to fill the blood vessels, which were dilating from the crisis.

Saline solution was ordered to fill up the volume.

Blood would have been better because saline solution doesn't transport oxygen the way red blood cells do. But no one even suggested this option.

For almost two hours the surgeons struggled with the crisis, alternately taking Mr. Hinden off the machine and putting him back on when he failed to respond. It took a long time but they would win this battle.

Finally, for reasons that are not clear to medical science, the heart started to respond. A fairly steady and effective beat, assisted by the balloon, began to replace the useless fibrillation.

The electrocardiogram pattern on the monitors improved.

The blood pressure climbed and the anesthesiologists could reduce the amount of drugs that were being pumped into Mr. Hinden. They could get him off the machine now.

"Okay, off the bypass and give him all the blood you've got," Dr. MacVaugh said.

"You've got it."

"Bottle the blood lines," Dr. MacVaugh ordered.

This was a critical decision. It would not be easy to turn back now. All the blood that had been pumping through the many tubes in the machine would be removed and put back into Mr. Hinden's body.

Because of his religious requirements they would not bottle the blood and drip it back to him. Instead, they hooked up a Rube Goldberg–type setup in which they hand-pumped the blood from the machine's lines into his blood vessels so that the continuity of the circulation wasn't broken.

For the first time in two hours the surgeons started talking to each other rather than barking out orders.

"Don't tell me you're quitting on us," Dr. MacVaugh said, kidding a nurse who was being replaced on this shift.

The tension was easing.

They had gotten Mr. Hinden off the machine, and all the readings looked fairly strong. They were still concerned that his badly scarred and weakened heart might be unable to survive the recuperative period. But there was nothing they could do about that. It was in someone else's hands now.

While Dr. Tomasello closed up the patient, Dr. MacVaugh went downstairs to his office to change into his street clothes and begin rounds.

On his way, he stopped by to talk to Mr. Hinden's wife, who had been waiting in the room outside the intensive-care unit all day.

It had stopped raining outside. The wet road glistened under the streetlamps and record low temperatures were turning the water into ice.

Dr. MacVaugh told Mrs. Hinden that her husband was still in danger, but that the surgery was over, and that he would soon come up to the intensive-care unit.

Mrs. Hinden thanked Dr. MacVaugh, who shook her hand and left for his rounds. But it would be a sad ending.

Two hours later Mr. Hinden died.

His heart stopped in the intensive-care unit.

Dr. Tomasello was with him when it happened. He opened up the chest right there and massaged Mr. Hinden's heart with his hands and shocked it with electricity.

They gave the drugs, and they gave the saline solution because they weren't allowed to give blood. For forty-five minutes they worked, trying to get the heart going again.

But it would not start, even with the aid of the balloon that was still pulsing inside the aorta.

The doctors did not know if the lack of blood made the difference. They certainly would have used several pints in both the operating room and the intensive-care unit if it hadn't been for Mr. Hinden's religion. But the ventricle was badly scarred, and no amount of blood would have corrected that.

Regardless of the cause, Mr. Hinden was dead.

But to the end, he had kept true to his faith.

25

It was early Monday morning and Lloyd and Jeannette Henderson were becoming increasingly concerned about Martha, their sick two-year-old daughter. She had slept an unusual amount over the weekend and still her fever refused to break.

The worried parents had no way of knowing it, of course, but Martha had a bacterial infection that would soon develop into meningitis, a serious inflammation of the lining of the spinal cord and brain. This would be particularly dangerous for Martha because she had sickle-cell anemia, a blood disease that, among other things, made it difficult to fight infections.

A comparatively minor infection in a person with sickle-cell anemia can turn into a serious, if not lethal, crisis if prompt and special care wasn't given. But the Hendersons didn't realize the dangers.

Hoping that a few more hours of rest would help, they let Martha sleep on.

□ □ □

The day shift was just arriving at Children's Hospital, or CHOP, as everyone called it. Because it was so early in the morning the normally hectic garden lobby was comparatively quiet.

The chairs in the McDonald's courtyard cafe, which later would be filled by squabbling children and harried parents, were now occupied by sleepy-eyed nurses and doctors fortifying themselves with gossip, coffee, and Egg McMuffins before starting the day.

Sitting at one of the tables was Mark Reber. He had been assigned to the hospital's hematology service, the specialized unit that dealt with blood diseases such as sickle-cell anemia.

Mark, who was now thirty, looked older than he had when he took his first clinical rotation at CHOP, only a year earlier. Flecks of gray were beginning to appear in his red beard.

He was sitting with Dr. Steven A. Shapiro and Dr. Judy C. Bernbaum, discussing the case of eleven-month-old Antonio Stefano, who had a mysterious bleeding problem that couldn't be diagnosed. All three were members of the hematology service, invariably called the heme team.

Antonio appeared healthy, but his stool was black, indicating the presence of blood, and his red-cell count, or hemoglobin, was low, a result of the bleeding problem. His unusually alert mother had brought him in because she, too, had had an undiagnosed blood problem.

"The hemoglobin is still around seven," Shapiro said. "By now I'd like to see it at around ten at least."

"The parents are asking about when they can go home," Mark said.

Shapiro nodded, knowing that the boy would have to stay in the hospital for another day of tests.

One possibility that had to be ruled out was hemophilia, a disorder in which the blood failed to clot properly and uncontrollable bleeding could occur, either internally or externally.

Finishing breakfast and throwing away the cups and plates, the heme team got up to begin the day. Dr. Shapiro and Mark would get the Stefano blood samples right after morning clinic, but they wouldn't get a chance to check them under the microscope until late in the afternoon.

Sickle-cell anemia was by far the most frequently encountered serious blood disorder at CHOP. Almost half of the hematology service's patients had this disorder, which occurred almost exclusively in blacks.

For reasons that were not clear, sicklers produced a lot of crescent-shaped red blood cells that had difficulty sliding through the smaller blood vessels the way normal oval-shaped red cells did.

Because of this, the cells frequently clogged the vessels, and the organs downstream of the blockage were without blood. Often, the result was terrible pain and tissue death.

One out of ten blacks was a genetic carrier of the sickle trait. The carriers had no symptoms of the disorder, but they ran a 25 percent chance of producing a sickle-cell-anemic child if the other parent also had the trait. One out of four hundred blacks had the disease.

Though there was no cure, modern medical techniques had made it possible for sicklers to live to their twenties and thirties, if not longer, instead of dying as infants or young children.

The best-informed expert on sickle-cell anemia at CHOP was Dr. Marie Oliveri Russell, thirty-two, an assistant professor of pediatrics at Penn. Dr. Russell was an attractive woman with a mischievous smile and the type of naturally messed-up, I-just-got-out-of-bed hair that less fortunate women spend a fortune to recreate in the beauty parlor.

Wearing a white plastic helmet to keep him from bumping his delicate head, three-year-old Jarvis Banks looked up angrily as Mark arrived to measure his swollen ankle and apparently paralyzed right leg. Jarvis was a hemophiliac.

Bleeding in the left side of his brain had weakened the right side of his body. Doctors weren't sure whether the stroke or the swollen ankle was responsible for Jarvis's inability to walk.

Mark greeted Jarvis with a smile and a hello, but the boy continued to glare at this red-bearded student in the white coat, who didn't seem to be there for his benefit.

Mark took out his little tape measure and handed it to Jarvis, but Jarvis wasn't interested.

"Here. You can play with this," Mark said.

"No!" Jarvis said. That was how he always replied when someone from the heme team questioned him.

Mark smiled. He was well accustomed to children, even uncooperative ones, having worked with emotionally disturbed children before entering medical school.

He pulled out the tape measure about a foot, held it in front of Jarvis's wide-open eyes and pushed the retract button.

"Poof!" he said as the tape vanished into its container.

Jarvis opened his mouth in surprise and Mark did it again. Then Jarvis reached out his hand for the magic instrument, and Mark gave it to him to play with.

As Jarvis played with the tape, Mark felt the boy's big belly and examined the leg.

Gently retrieving the tape, which Jarvis didn't want to relinquish, Mark measured his leg and ankle, noting the figures on his clipboard.

Then Mark got ready to leave, and Jarvis stared furiously at him for running away with his new toy. Playing the game, Mark stared just as intently back at Jarvis, displaying mock anger himself. Slowly, Jarvis's frown disappeared and a big smile brightened his face.

□ □ □

Most of the other patients visited by the team that morning had sickle-cell anemia. It was a terrible disease, causing many different problems for its young victims. The heme team was reminded of this daily as it made its rounds.

Angelina, a paper-clip-thin six-year-old child, had a low red blood cell count and a high fever. Because the sickle disease had lowered her immunity, infection was attacking her kidneys.

Harold, a twelve-year-old, had a heavy cast reaching past his waist. His hips had degenerated because the sickled cells had blocked the blood flow. Surgery had been needed to repair the damaged bone.

Vicki, a weary sixteen-year-old, had been brought into the hospital in excruciating pain a week earlier. She was in sickle-cell crisis caused by the disruption of blood flow to her joints and muscles. Now she had pneumonia, another complication of sickle-cell anemia.

And so it went on hematology rounds.

The members of the team were exhausted by the time they reached the hematology laboratory on the fifth floor. The preliminary report on the blood from Mrs. Stefano and her son was waiting for them.

The data were confusing.

The blood from both mother and son clotted normally, whereas hemophiliac blood takes an excessive time to clot. But other studies showed that both were deficient in Factor VIII the blood component needed for clotting.

Running her fingers through her wild hair, Dr. Russell studied the figures on the lab slips. Then she studied the blood under the microscope and asked other members of the team some questions.

After a long time she handed down her decision: "I'm betting it's von Willebrand's disease."

Von Willebrand's is a mild form of hemophilia that may lead to easy bruising or serious blood problems if the victim is not properly prepared for surgery, but usually is not fatal.

"I'll bet we'll find the disease running through the family," she said, turning to Mark. "Why don't you do a family tree on her?"

Mark nodded.

The next day he would sit down with Mrs. Stefano and ask her to remember as far back into her family as she could. Those persons who may have had a blood disorder would be identified and their relationship to Mrs. Stefano noted. If a pattern were found, it could help to identify the blood disorder.

The sun had just started to set by the time Mark got home for a night of reading up on blood disorders, von Willebrand's disease in particular.

□ □ □

That night, while Mark was studying his textbooks and Dr. Russell was tucking her own children into bed, a worried couple came into the CHOP emergency room. Lloyd and Jeanette Henderson were bringing in their daughter, Martha. Her fever was now up to 104 degrees.

A fever alone in a two-year-old was not normally something that worried pediatricians. The cause was usually a self-limiting virus infection that physicians couldn't do much about because viruses are immune to antibiotics.

But sicklers were treated differently because many complications were possible, and one of them was meningitis.

The Hendersons, unfortunately, neglected to tell the doctor on duty in the emergency room that Martha was a sickler.

After a brief examination, which failed to reveal meningitis or anything else serious, the doctor sent Martha and her parents home. The Hendersons were told to give Martha plenty of fluids and Tylenol, an aspirin substitute.

□ □ □

Mark had not even completed his third year at medical school, but already he and his classmates were worrying about what hospital they would train at after graduation the next year.

At the center of their concern was the immensely important dean's letter, which every student would receive. The letter is an evaluation of the student's medical and personal abilities, and in some ways it could be as important as the medical degree itself.

A very good evaluation virtually assured a Penn student of training at the hospital of his choice. A good hospital-training program would lead to good professional contacts, a better academic appointment if the student decided to go in that direction, or a more prestigious group practice. An unenthusiastic dean's letter might close some doors to the young doctor.

"Already it has started," Mark said, "the pressure making you worry about what residency program you will get into. They held a meeting of the class and explained how they were going to rank us compared to other classmates applying in the same field. You can't help thinking about that kind of stuff."

□ □ □

Mrs. Stefano was standing in the room, holding Antonio in her arms, when the heme team arrived Tuesday morning.

For five days, she had been sleeping on a cot next to her son's bed and she was anxious to go home.

Mark has been able to trace Antonio's family for three generations. He found that there appeared to be a pattern of bleeding disorders back to a great-grandfather who had died of a hemorrhage.

"We've got some of the results back on the blood test we've done on you and Antonio," Dr. Russell said to Mrs. Stefano, "and it seems very likely that Antonio has von Willebrand's disease."

The disease, named for Dr. Eric von Willebrand, the Finnish physician who identified it fifty years ago, sounded ominous. But Mrs. Stefano showed neither alarm nor fear. She stared at Dr. Russell and waited for her to continue.

Dr. Russell explained what the disease was and assured Mrs. Stefano that Antonio could lead essentially a normal life. He shouldn't be given aspirin, which could cause stomach bleeding, Dr. Russell said, and special preparations would be needed if he should require surgery or a tooth extraction.

All her life, Mrs. Stefano had known that something was wrong with her blood. Now it had been given a name and a doctor could tell her what to expect. The small dangers of the disease were turning out to be less threatening than the worries the unknown had conjured up.

As Dr. Russell explained, Mark and other members of the heme team stood in the background, listening and waiting to continue with their rounds.

Unlike many doctors who are primarily teachers, Dr. Russell maintained close contact with all of her patients during all phases of their stay. This was partly because of her personality and partly because of the nature of hematology—so much care was required over so long a period for victims of chronic blood disorders that even the highest-ranking doctors got to know their patients well.

Hematology was therefore somewhat frustrating for students and junior physicians because they did not have as much responsibility. On other services, the teaching doctors relied very much on the findings of the interns and even the students in assessing patients.

For a prospective physician, few things were as rewarding as contact with patients, especially the moments when he could go to a worried patient, explain what was wrong, and offer assurance that medical science would produce a solution.

In the hematology service, though, much of Mark's time was spent on more mundane duties, such as transcribing the dozens of laboratory blood readings from small slips of paper to larger pieces of paper and finally to the patient notebook.

At other times he would wait with the other members of the team to get a look on the double-view microscope as Dr. Russell explained the mysteries of the colorfully stained slides.

Mark elected hematology work because he planned to be a general pediatrician and believed it would be helpful to know about blood diseases.

But with the exception of sickle cell anemia, most of the blood diseases Mark had encountered were so rare that the general pediatrician rarely if ever saw them in the course of his practice.

At a referral hospital such as Children's, which got all the difficult cases the smaller hospitals couldn't handle, even the rarest disease appeared commonplace.

Tuesday was a quiet day.

A nine-year-old hemophiliac who would undergo surgery for a disfiguring blood clot on his face was prepared by the hematologists with an extra-large dose of blood components to assure clotting. Without them, he could bleed to death on the operating table.

Doctors in the intensive-care unit for infants requested a consultation on a five-day-old premature baby with a widespread infection. Using hands almost larger than the whole baby, Dr. Steven Shapiro stuck a hollow needle into the infant's back and drew a bone-marrow sample. It would be studied under the microscope to see if the child was able to make sufficient amounts of the blood components needed to fight infection.

□ □ □

The emergency call came to Dr. Shapiro on his pocket beeper as he was driving to the hospital early Wednesday morning. A dangerously ill patient had just come into the emergency room. They had difficulty arousing the child, and when they did she seemed unable to relate to her surroundings or the people around her. The presumptive diagnosis was meningitis. The emergency room doctor wanted help because she was a sickler.

The girl was Martha Henderson.

"On Tuesday she started slipping and falling when she tried to walk," Jeannette Henderson explained to Dr. Shapiro as he arrived at the emergency room.

"At first we thought she was having trouble with her shoes. But then she started shaking. When we came into her room this morning she was lying with her eyes open, staring at the ceiling. She didn't pay any attention to us. And her bottle was right next to her head. She hadn't touched it."

Lloyd Henderson stood next to his wife, looking at the floor, nodding in agreement. Martha was unconscious, curled up in the lap of an emergency room aide.

Dr. Russell came rushing down the hall to the emergency room, her long white coat flowing behind her. Dr. Shapiro briefed her on the case and Dr. Russell examined Martha, taking particular care to lift the child's head. The head resisted Dr. Russell's gentle lift.

It was a classic sign of meningitis. Infection had inflamed the child's spinal cord and brain. It hurt Martha to move her head. Even unconscious she resisted.

Four or five doctors were in the emergency room, each working on a different part of the unconscious child, who had been moved to an examining table.

Intravenous lines were put in to give her fluids and to provide huge amounts of antibiotics to wipe out the infection that had filled her blood. A general pediatrician listened to her heart. Two units of fluid, packed with red cells to help carry oxygen through the child's body, were made ready for transfusion.

The infectious disease specialists were notified and an isolation room was set aside on the fourth floor. As Martha was placed on a litter, Dr. Russell talked to the parents.

"This is a very serious infection to treat," Dr. Russell said, indicating without actually saying it that there was a very good chance it could kill their daughter.

She explained that the doctors would give Martha a lot of antibiotics, which were normally very effective in treating this infection, but added that children with sickle-cell anemia frequently did not respond well.

The mother did not cry at first, but a tear slid down her cheek as Dr. Russell spoke.

The fatality rate for sicklers with meningitis is 30 percent. Dr. Russell didn't mention that.

While the infectious disease specialists and other pediatricians worked on Martha through the afternoon and evening, the hematologists were busy examining the child's blood and spinal fluid to see whether her body was mounting an effective attack against the infection.

Bending down to the microscope, Dr. Shapiro focused on the spinal fluid sample. Hundreds of pepperlike specks jumped into focus as he went to high power. Normally the fluid is clear. The specks were bacteria that had invaded her spinal fluid.

Moving to the hematology laboratory, he looked at Martha's blood. Deformed crescent-shaped blood cells littered the field, clearly distinct from the normal oval-shaped blood cells.

The sickle cells were expected. He was more interested in seeing what kind of disease-fighting white cells were present in the blood and whether there were enough healthy red cells to carry oxygen.

The picture looked good. Dr. Shapiro saw a few white cells, two or three times bigger than the red cells, with a lot of granular material in them. These were leukocytes in the process of eating up the bacteria—a good sign.

Equally encouraging were the immature white cells he saw. Responding to the infection, Martha's bone marrow was producing white cells at such a rapid rate that it was pushing some of them into the bloodstream before they were mature.

The number of platelets, small blood components needed for clotting, was a little low, but there were enough of them to assure adequate clotting. And the hemoglobin level was high. Martha's immune system was forcefully fighting the infection.

With the aid of the antibiotics being dripped into her circulation, there was a good chance that she would make it, but she had a very difficult course ahead of her.

Martha's parents were huddled near the phone outside the isolation room when Dr. Shapiro reached the floor. He told them that things were progressing well. But he purposely did not give them a lot of encouragement at this point, saying that other doctors would talk to them later.

In the coming hours and days, the Hendersons came to understand on a very personal level why antibiotics were called the miracle drug.

Martha's response was dramatically swift.

By Thursday afternoon, the doctors could switch her to a general ward. She took nourishment and was alert enough to play with or at least touch a doll in her crib.

"She almost got up," her mother excitedly told Dr. Russell as the heme team came by on rounds. "She's moving about so good. And she's drinking a lot."

Dr. Russell agreed that that was good. But she told Mrs. Henderson that Martha still would have to be watched closely. Dr. Russell knew that Martha could easily take a turn for the worse, and she also was worried about possible brain damage.

Martha continued to improve, however. By Friday, she was alert and relating to people who played with her. Several days later she would go home.

□ □ □

The week was ending on a good note. It looked like Martha would be all right. Jarvis Banks's brain scan had showed the expected damage from the stroke, but there was no spread of the bleeding. Harold would be leaving for rehabilitation therapy soon. The doctors had succeeded in stopping Vicki's pain, and her pneumonia was being brought under control. Angelina's temperature had returned to normal and her kidneys were producing urine free of bacteria, indicating that the kidney infection had been brought under control.

The hematologists went home that week feeling good about how their specialty could control, if not cure, these serious blood disorders. But before Friday ended, the hospital admitted a teen-age girl with a pasty complexion and an alarming tendency to tire easily.

When the heme team looked at her blood under the microscope, they saw a slide cluttered with immature white cells with huge nuclei.

It was the unmistakable sign of leukemia—acute myelogenous leukemia, a type that responds poorly to treatment. The girl would be dead within the year.

Hematology—it is a specialty that sees a lot of tragedy.

26

He was a huge man with broad shoulders, a proud bearing, and deep penetrating eyes. He had come to the emergency room of the Presbyterian University of Pennsylvania Medical Center because of the bulging abscess under his left ear.

As he sat alone in a small treatment room waiting to be seen by a physician, he read *The Language of Feeling,* oblivious to those who walked by the open door.

It seemed incongruous for a big man such as he to be reading such a book in such a place, but, as the doctors would soon discover, this man did not fit the stereotype of someone this size.

Randy Wiest stood at the nurses' station, studying the man's admission papers. It looked as if it would be a simple, straightforward case, the kind he preferred.

Randy planned to enter family practice in a rural area after he graduated from medical school, and the four-week rotation in emergency room medicine was giving him his first opportunity to deal with the common medical problems he would see as a family doctor. Because of Penn's reputation, its teaching hospitals, such as Presbyterian, were most often filled with people suffering from complicated and unusual diseases.

The emergency room isn't a single room, but actually a dozen small examining and treatment cubicles off two corridors that bend around the nurses' station. It was particularly quiet this Thursday morning, probably because of the driving rain outside.

The more serious cases were kept in an open ward of six beds—with only curtains for privacy—so that the staff could easily keep an eye on patients who might suddenly need help. Hectic activity and noise usually dominated the emergency room, but it was quiet this morning; only the sound of the rain and the rock music on the ward clerk's radio disturbed the peace.

The few patients who had braved the storm sat by themselves in separate treatment rooms, waiting to be examined. Among them were a seventeen-year-old rape victim and a middle-aged woman with severe depression, a twenty-two-year-old man with sickle-cell anemia, a thirty-year-old man who had a stuffy nose from sniffing cocaine, and a man who had contracted gonorrhea from a woman who had insisted that she was free of disease.

As their cases show, the term *emergency room* is a misnomer. Less than one-fifth of the cases are true emergencies; most of the patients at Presbyterian's emergency room live in the surrounding west Philadelphia neighborhood, and their complaints are those that more affluent persons would take to their family doctor.

But most residents of urban ghettos are too poor to afford private care. For them, the emergency room is their family physician.

It is expensive and inefficient to treat mostly minor complaints with a facility staffed and equipped to provide costly emergency care. The service is rushed and impersonal and patients often must wait for hours, continually being bumped back on the waiting list by more urgent cases. But the people keep coming; their alternative is to go without any care at all.

On a busy day, Presbyterian's emergency room handles sixty to seventy patients.

Heavy rains kept patients away in the daytime, but brought them in at night because they did not have a dry place to sleep. In hot weather, asthmatics sat in the waiting room because the air-conditioning helped to relieve their symptoms. Regardless of what ails him, the street wise patient would tell the nurse that he had chest pains; he knew that this cardinal symptom of a heart attack would get him quicker care.

One of the slowest days of the month in the emergency room is the day the welfare checks arrived. Some people did not come in that day because they now had money to buy liquor; others did not come in because they had to guard their mailboxes against thieves.

"Got some bad news for you," an intern said to the man with veneral disease, who was listening impatiently because he already had recognized the symptoms.

"You got it, all right," the doctor continued. "That means no sex for two weeks."

"What?" the man said, his angry expression turning to one of alarm.

"Can't have you spreading that around," the intern said. "Got to give the drugs a chance to get rid of it."

"Okay, I'll be cool," the man said. "Don't feel much like it anyway, the way I feel now. Wait till I catch up with that . . ."

The big man put down the book when Randy came in with Dr. Karen Sharrar, a family practitioner and the director of the emergency room.

"What have we got here?" she said, going straight for the abscess, which Randy had examined and described to her.

"Yep," she said, feeling the lump between her fingers. The man winced.

Dr. Sharrar asked the man and Randy a few questions, poked around some more, and concluded that the abscess would have to be lanced. But she wanted a surgeon to perform the minor operation because the abscess was near the carotid artery, the main vessel feeding blood to the brain. A slight mistake with the scalpel could be fatal.

As Dr. Sharrar explained this to Randy, the man's eyes grew wider and filled with fear.

"There's something I've got to tell you," he said, grasping the closed book with his hands. "I'm scared of knives and needles and pain."

Dr. Sharrar looked surprised at what she had just heard from this giant of a man, and then a faint smile came to her face.

"We're not going to make you bite a bullet," she said touching his arm. "We'll give you something for the pain."

The man shook his head sighing. "There's just no way I like those knives, just no way."

□ □ □

Randy was enjoying his rotation in the emergency room. It was giving him the sense of confidence that had been lacking ever since he started his hospital rotations. Most of the cases in the emergency room were simple enough so that Randy could deal with them on his own, without constantly going to someone above him for advice.

Randy was discovering that all he had learned in the lectures halls, laboratories, and the other rotations did amount to a significant mass of knowledge—enough knowledge to treat most of the patients likely to come into the emergency room. After so many months of self-doubt and feelings of insecurity as a student, the emergency room experience was reassuring for Randy just as it would be for Rikki Lights and just as it was for most students who took the rotation.

Much of emergency room medicine consisted of checking people to make sure that they didn't have something that could or should be treated and then reassuring them that everything would probably be all right. Office practice medicine largely consisted of that type of work, which was fine with Randy because he liked relating to patients as much if not more than doing the diagnostic and therapeutic procedures.

Students like Matt Lotysh found such medicine mundane and boring and headed for the dramatic life-and-death medicine of the cardiovascular surgeon. Conversely Randy found cardiovascular surgery tedious because it was more involved in technique and technology than relating. That was one reason Randy would work for two years as a U.S. Public Health Service physician in a rural area after he completed his internship. One plan was to go to Alaska, where he could combine family practice medicine with his love of the outdoors.

Even in the third year, Randy wasn't sure that he liked medicine. He was still reserving judgment because he hoped that office practice medicine was different from academic medicine, which he knew he didn't like. Academic medicine was too high pressured. The people were too impersonal. And he himself didn't have time to relate to people either. One day during a pause in the emergency room activity, Randy confessed some of his concern to an acquaintance.

"I don't know," he said, looking at a ward clerk filling out the chart of a patient who had just arrived, "but maybe it's just the stage of training I'm in. I'm so busy worrying about relating to people's physical problems that I don't have a chance to relate to them in other than the most superficial way. I try to take account of their feelings and where they are emotionally. But the nature of the short-term interaction I have with a patient just doesn't add up to anything."

Randy was also missing his wife, Marge. She had finally decided to drop out of medical school for a year and had gone to Virginia to teach science to high school students. They'd see each other on occasional weekends, but the distance of geography and careers was disturbing.

It was possible that Marge might leave medicine altogether. If she decided to return, she'd be a year behind her husband. This wouldn't constitute a major problem because she could finish her fourth year wherever Randy went for internship training. But still the third year of medical school was turning out to be difficult for Randy and Marge on both personal and professional levels.

□ □ □

The surgeon who would lance the abscess came down, dressed in a green scrub suit. The big man awaited the impending procedure with terror, but to the surgeon it was a trifle that was taking him away from more important things.

Steadily talking to Randy and the emergency room intern as he worked, the surgeon quickly confirmed the need for lancing. He told the big man to lie on a treatment table and filled the hypodermic syringe with a pain-killing drug.

"What's the matter?" the surgeon said, surprised that his unwilling patient had pulled his head back. "This is just a little needle."

He injected the little needle into the man's skin, and the big man groaned loudly.

Ignoring the man and talking to Randy as the drug took effect, the surgeon cleaned the area where he would operate. Then he got a scalpel and cut into the abscess.

"Yow" the big man screamed, so loudly that Dr. Sharrar rushed in to see what was happening. "Oh, my God," he moaned, kicking his legs into the plastic curtain that separated the treatment room from an adjoining one.

"Hey, where are you going?" the surgeon said. "You can't go into the next room because that's a pediatric unit for children." He laughed at his joke. No one else did.

Several times more the big man screamed out in pain, although the surgeon moved swiftly and completed the process in a matter of minutes.

"See, that didn't hurt so much," the surgeon said to the still moaning patient.

□ □ □

By early afternoon, the rain had stopped and the pace began to pick up in the emergency room.

A ring had to be cut off the swollen finger of a woman who had hurt her hand when she hit her boyfriend in the face. A huge highway patrolman complained of a nosebleed; an intern cauterized his nose to stop the bleeding as a fellow patrolman stood guard outside the treatment room. It was a painful procedure, but the policeman did not flinch once, maintaining a stoic, machismo posture.

A woman who weighed well over two hundred and fifty pounds was wheezing so badly she could barely stand. She was placed in the large treatment room and given drugs to ease her breathing.

A man with a disjointed finger came in. Dr. Sharrar asked him what was wrong. Without saying a word, he merely stuck the crooked finger in Dr. Sharrar's face.

Smiling, she grabbed the finger and yanked it straight. The suddenness of the treatment astonished the man, who winced in momentary pain.

Another man came in with an aching wisdom tooth. Someone else had been bitten by a dog. Two more cases of venereal disease were treated and another rape victim was brought in and taken to a private treatment room.

There were a few colds, a couple of drunks, and someone who had such a bad case of itching hemorrhoids that he could not sit down.

The most interesting case of the day turned out to be the seventeen-year-old boy who came in with a bulge in his groin. He had recently been treated for a stab wound in this area. The bulge might have been a complication.

"There's definitely a bruit," Randy said to Dr. Sharrar after examining the boy. As she placed her stethoscope on the bulge, the embarrassed teenager tried to use his hands to shield his exposed genitals.

"Some third-year surgical resident is going to be very interested to see this," Dr. Sharrar said.

The bruit—a noise they heard through the stethoscope—meant that blood was rushing through the bulge, an indication that the problem was definitely not a minor one.

The most fearful possibility was that the stabbing had nicked and weakened an artery, which then had ballooned like a defective inner tube and was now about to blow out. If it did, the boy could bleed to death in minutes.

Once again the surgeon came down to the emergency room, but this time he was much more interested. His examination took only minutes.

"We've got to operate right away," the surgeon said. He thought a major blood vessel was ready to burst. "Let's get him ready to go upstairs."

Within minutes the youth's room was filled with aides and nurses. An intravenous tube was prepared. A nurse shaved the boy's abdomen. An electrocardiogram was taken and studied to make sure his heart could stand the stress of surgery without special precautions.

The youth was dumbfounded by the activity. He had come in with a bulge and assumed that a little medicine and a few bandages would take care of it. But now all this was happening around him. He just kept swinging his head left and right like a frightened rabbit, afraid of the slightest movement.

"Do you have someone you want us to notify?" said an aide with a big clipboard in her hand.

"Huh?" the boy said.

"Your mother? Your father?"

"Huh?"

"Do you know you're being admitted to the hospital?"

The boy shook his head.

"Do you know we're taking you to surgery?"

The boy's eyes and mouth opened wider, but all he could do was once again shake his head.

□ □ □

Kate Treadway replaced Randy as the student on duty at 4:00 P.M. The seventeen-year-old was still in surgery. Once again the emergency room had become quiet, and the staff took advantage of the unusual calm to talk about vacations past and future.

At 5:10 a man came in with a gouge in his arm. His girl friend had attacked him with a sharp-heeled shoe. It had apparently been a big fight; she followed him into the emergency room holding a bandage over a black eye.

Dr. Sharrar was gone now, and a moonlighting internal medicine fellow from the HUP, Dr. William Follansbee, had taken her place. A young, well-groomed man, he dressed with spiffy formality and spoke with the literate completeness of a Princeton graduate, which he was.

Kate had just finished working on an alocholic woman who was complaining of stomach pain. Kate's examination failed to reveal anything unusual, and she did not think the woman's problem was serious. Dr. Follansbee did not agree with Kate's conclusion.

"A lot of people tend to do less on this type of patient," Dr. Follansbee said, meaning a drunk with no clear-cut problem, "but I like to do more with them just because of that fact."

It seemed to make sense. Because of their drinking, alcoholics are prone to many medical problems, but a lot of doctors tend to be less sympathetic toward self-induced illness. Not Dr. Follansbee.

Walking into the examining room with Kate in tow, Dr. Follansbee proceeded to give the thin little woman with the painful stomach an extensive interview and examination.

"Do you have mucus in your bowel movements? Has the volume increased?" he asked.

"What?" the woman said, slurring her words, confused by all the questions.

"Have your legs been swelling?"

"Yes."

"How long?"

"Since I've had children."

"Do you have diabetes?"

The woman looked confused. "Huh?" she asked.

"Do you have trouble with your sugar?"

"Yes."

"Ah," Dr. Follansbee said, pleased with the success of his translation.

Abruptly disengaging from the woman, Dr. Follansbee asked Kate: "What's the next question when they say they have trouble with their sugar?"

"Do you take insulin?" Kate said tentatively.

"I'll tell you something," the woman said, reacting to the enthusiasm over her case, "when I put a bruise on myself it stays there."

"Oh," Dr. Follansbee said. "Do you eat well?"

"Of course I do."

"What do you eat?"

"A lot of beans and potatoes and cabbage," she said.

"How much do you drink?"

"Hey, look," the woman said, getting defensive now, "my drinking has nothing to do with my problem."

"You sure?" Dr. Follansbee asked.

"I want a cigarette," she said, apparently losing interest in the questions.

After asking a few more questions, Kate and Dr. Follansbee retreated to the corridor, closing the door behind them. Dr. Follansbee was sure that the woman's severe dietary deficiencies could account for her problem. Once the precise deficiencies were determined he could tell the woman what corrective measures could be taken.

Dr. Follansbee asked Kate to suggest some appropriate tests, offered several more suggestions himself, and told her to get them done.

First they got an x-ray of the woman's chest. She didn't like it because she had to stand up and remain still for so long.

And they stuck her with needles to get blood tests for this thing and that. She didn't like the needles either and couldn't understand why they were doing all these things to her.

She began to get mad. She wanted to smoke a cigarette, but there was no place in the emergency room where this was permitted. Finally she persuaded the doctors to allow her to smoke a cigarette in the waiting room until they were ready to give her the next test in the extensive battery that Dr. Follansbee had outlined to Kate.

It was a long wait, but finally the technicians were ready for the woman. They went out to the waiting room to get her. But she was gone.

The good doctors hadn't tired of the tests, but she had.

The evening dragged on, and the complaints were minor. A cold. A cut on the chin. A headache from high blood pressure. Things picked up a bit at 8:50 P.M., when the police brought in a father and son who had both been stabbed in a fight with another son.

Stabbings always tied up the emergency room. The doctors had to perform an especially careful examination to ensure that nothing serious has been damaged. Closing the wound itself involved time-consuming stitching. And in serious cases, a lot of standby preparations had to be made in case the patient's blood loss caused his blood pressure to drop to the point of bringing on shock and possibly a heart attack.

The injured son had received chest wounds, and air was building up in his chest cavity outside the lungs. The doctors had to put a tube in to let the air out and make arrangements to hospitalize him. A priest arrived to reassure the two victims. "It's a real Cain and Abel situation," he said to a doctor, who nodded without replying.

At 11:10 Kate's evening was ruined. A young boy came in with a knee injury, and x-rays revealed a broken bone. Kate had seen the boy the night before and, with the approval of the intern, had sent him home without x-rays she should have ordered because the injury seemed minor. But the pain had grown worse, so the boy was brought back.

"These things happen to everyone," Dr. Follansbee reassured Kate, who kept berating herself for the mistake. "This is a good lesson for you. That's why it's so important to be extra careful in the emergency room. A lot of times you don't get a second chance like you do in private practice, when you have a continuing relationship with your patients. If you miss it here on the first contact, they might leave, and you will not get a second chance."

Kate nodded her head sadly as he spoke.

"Oh, I feel so terrible," she said.

It was past midnight now, time for Kate to go home. Only the moans of a jogger disturbed the quiet of the emergency room. Kate and the doctors were intrigued with his case because he was a diagnostic mystery. He had been suddenly striken with sharp stomach pains while running.

The fat asthmatic woman was breathing better now, and a cab had been called for her. Someone was being admitted with a cut on his palm. Once again the staff could hear the rock and roll music on the little radio.

All told, sixty-four people had been treated in the emergency room since Randy had come on duty at 8:00 A.M. Venereal disease. Two rapes, two stabbings. A lot of colds and back pains and stomach pains and one broken jaw. Even some emergency surgery—the boy's blood vessel had been succesfuly repaired. It had turned out to be a busy day, considering the slow start during the rain.

None of the cases were particularly dramatic, but all were very important to the patients.

Kate finally left for home at 12:30 in the morning. It would be some time before the doctors found out what was wrong with the big man with the stomach pain.

But that was for the next shift.

When Kate joined her husband at home she would not be talking about the jogger anyway. She would be telling her husband about the little boy who had come in the night before with a hurt knee and how she had sent him home without an x-ray.

27

The months in Virginia had been good ones, and Marge Shamonsky was happy that she had made the decision to leave medical school for a while.

She was teaching marine biology to high school students at a marine science station in Chincoteague, and she had also been doing some work in a medical clinic twenty miles to the south in Onley, Virginia.

It was good to get outdoors again. She had forgotten how much she enjoyed the life and work. Medical school seemed a million miles and a hundred years away. Every few weeks she would see Randy and he would bring her up to date on what was happening in the world she had been so glad to leave. There was no nostalgia, no feelings of loss for this world, no yearning to return. She in turn would tell Randy about what it was like working in the clinic, where most of the medical problems were straightforward and one doctor stayed with the case from the beginning to the end rather than passing the patient down a line of specialists. And Randy would again feel good about the prospects for a medical career and feel strong in his decision to become a family practitioner, probably practicing in a rural area not unlike Onley.

Marge had come to admire the doctor in the clinic and the way he related to his patients. She liked socializing with him and the other people in the clinic and the people in the marine science station. It was not like that at medical school, where the socializing was almost zero and all the talk was about medicine.

As the months passed, Marge realized that she would soon have to determine whether or not to return to medical school. It was becoming an increasingly difficult decision because the fresh, good memories of relating to people in Virginia were making the old memories of medical school so much bleaker by comparison.

She remembered the intern who got annoyed when relatives wanted to talk to him about the woman who had just died of aplastic anemia. And she remembered the painful hours spent at cafeteria tables with residents who refused to talk to her, a mere student. And the lonely nights at home while Randy was on call at a hospital. And the crowded dirty city and the growing feelings of worthlessness that came from always being ignored.

She didn't want to return to that world, not after finding her self-esteem again in Virginia. But even with all these thoughts, it was not easy to give up the plan to become a physician.

She had worked so hard to get into medical school in the first place, beating the three-to-one odds.

She would be throwing away a chance most people didn't get. And she had invested two years of very hard work in medical school already. If she left now she would leave with nothing, but if she stuck it out for only another two years, at least she would have a medical degree to show for her labors.

But then her thinking would seesaw back again to the other side of the argument. It wasn't just a matter of finishing another two years of medical school. She'd also have to work an absolute minimum of one year in the hospital as an intern just to get a license, and she would probably end up doing a couple years of residency training on top of that.

An important consideration that finally swayed Marge was the thought of money—not the money she would earn as a physician, but the indebtedness she had accumulated already as a medical student. She was up to $15,000 in debt and it would come due when she left medical school. The thought of paying back such a large amount on a teacher's salary was disturbing. And there were still many specialized areas of medicine that she would like to investigate, like rehabilitation medicine, where teams of people worked closely together with patients. And, of course, there was the good experience she had had in the Onley clinic. If she could find a career like that it would be rewarding, perhaps enough to make all of the pain of medical school worthwhile.

Finally Marge decided to return to Philadelphia in December. She would complete her third year of medical school at Penn and for the fourth year go to whatever school was in the area Randy went to for his residency training.

Since Randy disliked the city as much as she did, she knew it would be in a more rural or scenic area than Philadelphia. That thought, at least, made the prospects of returning more bearable as the final months in Virginia slipped away.

□ □ □

During the third year, as they became more accustomed to their roles in the hospital, the students also became more critical of medicine in general and academic medicine in particular. The biggest complaint was that it was so impersonal on both a doctor/patient level and doctor/student level. The rare cases that were attracted to centers like HUP and associated hospitals were beginning to annoy the students because they knew such a patient population wouldn't be encountered in the average practice.

Deborah Spitz was becoming increasingly annoyed at the way the field of psychiatry was continually being put down by the physicians at the HUP.

One day she was sitting in the HUP cafeteria with a friend who was chiding her about clinging to her dream of becoming a psychiatrist.

"You're too good at medicine to go into a field like psychiatry," he said.

Deborah looked at him sharply.

"I mean, what good do shrinks do?" he persisted. "It's a worthless field."

"What do you mean?" Deborah shot back. "You think medicine is so much more worthwhile? You think it's so worthwhile to watch a diabetic for ten years and not be able to do that much for him? You think monitoring the progress of a disease you can't treat is really doing something? You can be very busy monitoring diabetes. And monitoring coronary artery disease. And monitoring cancer. Most of medicine is monitoring the progress of inevitable disease processes. We can cure surgical problems. We can cure infectious diseases. But the rest of it we watch."

Her friend just sat looking at her. He was dumbfounded by the attack, unaware that Deborah was releasing anger that had been building up for a long time.

He was about to change the subject, but Deborah wasn't through.

"Most of you people who go into medicine are exactly the kind of people who can't deal with uncertainties and vagueness," she continued. "You're all so obsessive. You like to count things. You like things that are exact. Psychiatry is too vague for you. You want something you can measure. You people are so damned scared of something that isn't quantifiable."

Deborah became silent. She was finished. It felt good to have let it out.

"Hey, did you see *Roots* on TV last night?" her friend asked.

□ □ □

Steve Levine had thought that the most rewarding part of medicine would be dealing with patients, but after almost three years of medical school and two years in the hospitals he was becoming disappointed.

Most of Steve's classmates disagreed, but Steve thought there was an unusual number of hostile patients, especially in places like the emergency room. He was talking about it one day to an associate outside the operating rooms where he was doing a rotation.

"In the emergency room, before you can introduce yourself to the patient, they come over to you and scream at you and yell," Steve said. "You work and work and work over the patient and you get absolutely no gratitude, no recognition, just hostility, just suspicion, just negative vibrations. It's very easy to see how doctors start calling patients turkeys or crocks or psych cases."

An intern sat down with Steve and the other student and listened. No one got a chance to speak because, like Deborah, he had been storing these feelings up for a long time and wanted to let them all out.

"I've taken all this hostile crap just wandering around as a poor little medical student, more than I ever did as a psychologist. I've seen more psychotics and homicidal maniacs and just plain hostile people trying to sew a cut on a finger than I would have if I went out looking for it. I have to decide how much of that I'm going to take before I go into a primary care specialty. Hospital medicine is a lot of 'us' against 'them'—the intern stonewalling down in the emergency room, trying to keep the patients out to protect their friends upstairs who don't want more patients."

Medical school was taking its toll on Steve. He was developing some bitterness—not only about the patients but low-level hospital employees who tried to avoid work and inefficient hospitals that used medical students as cheap labor, and the lack of intellectual excitement in the profession, which, at his level at least, seemed dominated by endless repetitive work like getting lab results and drawing blood.

Also his marriage was breaking up. There had been problems before medical school, but the stress of the long hours undoubtedly had contributed to its collapse.

□ □ □

Matt Lotysh was in a comparatively good space, putting all his energies into his work and into surgery, ignoring the other problems that were confronting students who wanted more out of their lives now than just medicine.

Matt was very discouraged after his second year and he left Penn to spend the summer working at the Milton S. Hershey Medical Center in rural Hershey, Pennsylvania. This was the hospital for the Pennsylvania State University College of Medicine.

Matt had been worn out by the grind at the HUP and he wanted freedom and relaxation. He learned how to play tennis in Hershey and he met a lot of nice women and he rediscovered the other things in life that were worthwhile. But unlike students such as Randy Wiest and Marge Shamonsky he found them lacking.

Hershey simply was not aggressive enough for someone like Matt Lotysh. The thing that he wanted to escape from—the competition and the continuous demand for more and better work—was the very thing Matt liked and wanted. He didn't realize it until he escaped from it to languish in the unpressured atmosphere of a less demanding institution.

He knew that at Penn the more the student proved himself and the more he pushed to get responsibility, the more the staff would allow him to do. The type of medicine that turned Randy off turned Matt on—the big, the daring, the competitive.

So Matt was like a hungry animal when he returned to Penn. His rotation through cardiothoracic surgery under Dr. MacVaugh at the start of the third year couldn't have been better timed.

His leisure in Hershey had primed him for the demanding rotation. He ate it up, staying on duty for twelve, fourteen, eighteen hours at a time, when no one expected or suggested that he should. But it didn't matter, because this was the one place in the world he most wanted to be in—even more than going out with the nurses who always seemed attracted to him.

On the nonsurgical rotations, Matt seemed almost disinterested. He did his work adequately and passed the courses but without particular distinction, almost as though he was saving his energies for the surgery.

More than anyone else in the class, Matt exemplified the compulsive, hard-driving, competitive medical student.

□ □ □

Ron Cargill spent much of the third year struggling with his conscience. All along he had intended to go into general medicine so he could practice medicine in the ghetto and help the black people. But he was coming to dislike general medicine. So much of it involved patients with chronic disease that could not be effectively treated. It was frustrating, if not depressing.

Ron found new enthusiasm, however, in anesthesiology. It was an exciting field with so many different aspects that were interesting. During the preoperative period, the anesthesiologist related closely to the patients at a time when they were scared and needed support. When the surgery started, the anesthesiologist was called upon to be extremely alert because anesthetics were tricky and could easily kill if administered carelessly. And after surgery the anesthesiologist was the primary physician responsible for pulling the patient through the difficult hours of recovery. The modern anesthesiologist was gaining an increasingly strong role in the intensive-care units, where his knowledge about respiration, airways, and drugs circulating through the body was so important.

Anesthesiology was critical care medicine, and Ron liked knowing that what he did as an anesthesiologist could make a major difference in the outcome of the case. In fact, it could have life-and-death consequences.

He spoke about his thoughts of changing career goals with his advisers at Rutgers University, who were black. And they were disappointed. They felt the need was to get black doctors into the community, where they could not only treat their black brothers and sisters but serve as role models to the world—showing that blacks were making their way in the prestigious sectors of society. Ron argued that there were few black anesthesiologists but that there were a lot of black surgical patients who could benefit from a black anesthesiologist.

It sounded like a reasonable argument, but Ron's advisers weren't accepting the rationale. Ron wasn't too comfortable with it either. He would think about it some more. He had dedicated himself to helping his people, but anesthesiology was so exciting. Ron found it as exciting as he had found general medicine discouraging.

In the third year, Jim Nestor began to think like a doctor rather than an engineer. Biology was too complex and medical science too imperfect to work things out from first principles, as an engineer does. Jim was now thinking in terms of differential diagnoses. This is a process whereby a physician makes a diagnosis by comparing the patient's symptoms with dozens of syndromes or clusters of symptoms associated with specific diseases. It didn't so much require abilities in deductive reasoning as it did a very good eye and an even better memory.

After his disappointing experience with pediatrics, Jim started seeking another career goal. He was becoming particularly interested in three different specialties for sharply different reasons.

He liked epidemiology because it required the mind of a detective working out a mystery, and it was a field where a lot of good could be done. Stopping or limiting one epidemic could prevent more disease and death than a dozen doctors might in a lifetime.

Cardiology was also interesting to Jim because it appealed to his engineering mentality. As Jim saw it, the heart was nothing more than a pump, and what cardiology required was knowledge of fluid mechanics.

And finally he liked radiology because he was good at it. Again his training as an engineer made it easier for him than most other students to look at two-dimensional x-ray films and visualize what they represented in three dimensions.

Jim was becoming much more a part of the medical profession. Not only was he thinking more like a physician, he was beginning to get a better understanding of the physician's problems.

The long hours and endless work and the army of patients encountered in a teaching hospital made it difficult continuously to think of the human factors. He hoped that this was just a phase of the training. He had to concentrate on the mechanics of medicine because he was so unsure of himself. Like Randy, he couldn't deal with the patient's anxiety and other emotional needs as much as he would like. Perhaps from the outside, he thought, it appeared that he was crass. But he just didn't know enough to discuss their problems at length. And there just wasn't enough time.

Jim Nestor was not in a comfortable space.

The third year of medical school was psychologically important in that it was past the halfway point. The students knew that they had less work before them than they had already done. They had no longer to fear surprises. They had fallen into the routine and had become comfortable in their role as students working with patients in a hospital.

Though they had their disappointments and discouragements with medicine, the anxiety was gone now. In a way they were coasting toward the next hurdle in their careers—finding a hospital to do postgraduate work in as an intern or first-year resident. In the fourth year all their energies and thoughts would be devoted to these questions: "Where will I match? What hospital will accept me for my training?"

But for the present, in this their third year, the students thought only of their rotations and the tedium and the hard work. It was no longer painful. But the romance of medicine had begun to fade.

28

Rikki Lights tried to conceal her anxiety by joking with a fellow student as they waited in the obstetrics unit at Pennsylvania Hospital.

"If I drop that baby," Rikki said with a flash of her long fingers for emphasis, "I'm dropping this course."

In a few hours the twenty-four-year-old student would, for the first time, deliver a baby.

Rikki sat at a long bank of cluttered desks. Here in a large windowless room the doctors and nurses filled out charts and did other clerical work while waiting for the women in labor to give birth.

A dozen doors led off of this room to cubicles where big-bellied women struggled with the last hours of labor, aided by nurses and pain-deadening drugs. To the rear were the swinging doors of the delivery rooms.

The moaning of a sixteen-year-old girl came from one of the rooms. She was fighting the contractions and this made the pain worse. She didn't know better, even though this was her second pregnancy.

From another room came a synthetic *tap-tap* sound—the amplified beat of a fetal heart, transmitted by an ultrasonic device strapped to the distended belly of a woman.

This particular woman was only five feet tall, yet tests indicated that the baby she was about to deliver weighed nearly ten pounds. There was concern that the baby would not be able to pass through the woman's pelvic opening and that a Caesarean section would have to be performed.

It was 12:30 in the afternoon. One of the "ladies," as the patients were called in the obstetrics unit, would deliver shortly and either Rikki or Elaine Wilson, twenty-four, another third-year student, would assist.

It did not matter who went first because both students would get their chance. They were on call, which meant they would work straight through the night until 7:00 the next morning.

With more than three thousand births a year, Pennyslvania averaged eight babies a day. Rikki and Elaine would get plenty of experience this shift.

□ □ □

The four-year education that turns a layman into a physician is dotted with symbolic milestones—the first patient, the first physical examination and laying on of hands, the first cadaver, the first operation, the first autopsy.

Each experience, with all its intense emotions, slightly transformed the student so after a while he no longer thought and felt and saw things in quite the same way as nondoctors.

It was in this way that a layman became a physician.

And of all the milestones, none was more moving or awesome than the experience of delivering a baby for the first time. The emotional impact of watching a new life begin was as intense as watching an old one end.

Most Penn medical students took obstetrics even though they were not required to and professionally would never have need to know how it was done. Obstetrics was an elective course, and most Penn graduates went into specialties like surgery, internal medicine, and psychiatry.

Obstetrics was considered a happy specialty. A lot of students chose it because of this. But it also had excitement. Probably no other branch of medicine had experienced as many scientific and technological advances in the last decade as had obstetrics—especially perinatology, the medical discipline that covered the period just before, during, and after birth.

□ □ □

"I think I felt something hard," Rikki said, coming out of a labor room. She had just measured the cervical opening of a woman about to give birth, feeling with the fingers of her gloved hand.

"That was the baby's head," said Dr. Jeffrey I. Scharf, a friendly, easygoing, second-year obstetrical resident.

"Oh," Rikki said, a little embarrassed.

Dr. Scharf was peering at an illuminated x-ray film. It showed the pelvis of the woman whose smallness was a concern. Measuring the opening shown on the film with a ruler, Dr. Scharf compared it with the baby's skull, now only a few inches away from the birth canal. It looked as if it would be a very tight fit.

A Caesarean section, or C-section, as the doctors called it, was not especially dangerous, but obstetricians did not want to do one unless they had no choice.

Because of the weakening of stomach muscles due to the incision to remove the baby, performing a C-section on the woman usually condemned her to this method of birth for all future pregnancies, with all the attendant annoyances and risks of anesthesia, wound infection, and increased length of stay in the hospital.

No, it would be better to wait a little longer before making a decision. The woman was in good labor and the ultrasonic monitor indicated a strong steady fetal heart rate. The baby's pulse dipped only momentarily when the fetus was squeezed by the pressure of a contraction, but the rate rose again quickly.

Dr. Scharf told Rikki how to measure a pelvic opening and then disappeared, leaving her to wait for the delivery in which she would assist.

It would be a little while; a coin toss had determined that the first delivery would go to Elaine.

Rikki sat down at the nurses' station and started reading the textbook on obstetrics, trying to ignore the periodic cries of pain from the sixteen-year-old in labor.

At 1:33 P.M., Elaine assisted in the delivery of the first baby. With a resident giving her step-by-step instructions, Elaine eased a bluish white baby into the world. The baby cried immediately and required comparatively little suctioning to clear the airways of fluid.

Throughout the procedure, Rikki watched from the sidelines, trying to remember just how Elaine had turned the infant as it came out to help the shoulders through the narrow opening.

It hadn't seemed particularly difficult.

Rikki returned to the nurses' station to wait. The next delivery was hers.

□ □ □

Rikki was still not happy about medicine. She had not found the art and now wondered more than ever if there was an art, a creativity, to it.

She continued to stay by herself, but knew that her being different was working to her disadvantage. Even on this rotation she was beginning to pick up negative vibrations because she didn't seek extra work but preferred to go home and do her writing.

Many of the doctors around her were jealous of her creativity and the breadth of her interests. And Rikki wasn't very tactful. She didn't pretend interest or adulation the way many of her classmates did.

The word had gotten out that she had married someone with end-stage renal disease and a lot of people were wondering out loud why anyone would marry someone with a terminal illness. It annoyed Rikki because the criticism suggested that someone with renal disease had nothing to offer but the pathology.

Rikki was also under a lot of pressure because some doctors in obstetrics were annoyed at her diverse interests. Rikki was a character and it was difficult for the straight doctors to accept this. She dressed in a dramatic style, was interested in the world of art, and wasn't very good at playing the academic game.

Rikki felt that they were demanding that she be like them or else they would reject her. She confessed her fears to a friend one night in the staff lounge in the obstetrics unit:

"They want something that I can't give them," she said. "They want me to adopt their lifestyle. But I think that medicine is independent of lifestyle. I insist that medicine is apart from all this hazing. And that's what it is—hazing. I don't want to live like these people. I don't want to live in constant fear and terror without love or compassion or knowledge or anything outside myself. I've looked carefully at their value system and I've decided that there is a good portion of it I don't want. It's the white academia value system. It's white elitism. It's white maleism. Maleness. Detachment. It's worse at Penn than at Bryn Mawr."

Her friend agreed. Her friend was a black, woman, medical student.

□ □ □

Between deliveries, an uneasy calm settled over the obstetrics unit. It was something like a firehouse, with everyone whiling away the time by doing odd jobs until the next alarm sounded.

Some of the nurses waited in the central desk, chatting, while others sat in the cubicles with the expectant mothers, monitoring their labor. Every now and then a physician or student would go to one of the women, don a glove, and measure the opening of her cervix with his fingers. When it reached ten centimeters the cervix was fully dilated and the birth was only thirty minutes to an hour away.

This prompted a flash of activity. Nurses wheeled the patient into the delivery room. The woman was switched to the delivery table and made ready. Doctors, nurses, and students scrubbed at the sink. Then the moment of delivery. And then there was the return to the uneasy calm.

Frequently the babies came so fast the deliveries overlapped, and then there was a constant stir of activity. But this day had been quiet at Pennsylvania Hospital, and Rikki had nothing to do but wait, while Elaine filled out the sheaf of papers making the baby's birth official.

Sitting there, Rikki surveyed all the sophisticated devices and the varied staff of doctors, nurses, and aides. Rikki recalled a recent visit to her home in Sea Island, South Carolina, and reflected that if there were serious complications, a mother and her baby would fare much better in a place like Pennsylvania Hospital.

Rikki's reverie was broken by an awareness of hushed activity in the corner of the large windowless room. Several physicians had come out of the room of the small woman and were huddled outside of her door.

They had just broken the woman's water bag to start the birth process, and the fluid was brownish. The cause was meconium—a fetal bowel movement.

Meconium is a danger signal. A fetus makes meconium only when it's under stress. The physicians did not know what the stress was but they were afraid to allow it to continue for fear that it might damage the fetus. They were also concerned that the additional stress of the birth process would cause the unborn baby to breathe in the bowel movement floating in the fluid of the amnionic sac. This could damage the lungs and possibly kill the baby.

The baby must be delivered quickly with a C-section, the doctors decided.

For a moment it looked as if Rikki's first baby would be an obstetrical emergency. But before the C-section could be started, another woman completed the final stages of her labor and was quickly wheeled to a delivery table.

Dr. Sharf entered the room and nodded to Rikki. She smiled, got up and began preparing for the delivery.

Most births are without complications, and about all the physician has to do is catch the infant as it comes out. But this very basic process is made to appear unnatural, almost like a surgical procedure, by all the preparations that are made to guard against a mishap.

The woman is shaved and draped with green surgical sheets. Her legs are strapped into stirrups, raising her legs in an ungainly position higher than her head. And the expressions on all the faces around are hidden by green masks, leaving only the eyes to transmit unspoken feelings.

"You help the head out by pulling on the chin," Dr. Scharf said to Rikki as the two of them scrubbed and rescrubbed their hands at the sink in the hallway outside of the delivery room. Now they were both wearing masks and conductive paper booties to contain dirt and prevent static electricity from igniting gas in the operating room.

"Turn the baby as it comes out," Dr. Scharf continued. "This will help the shoulders get out."

Rikki was listening without saying anything as the two kept scrubbing. It really was not a very difficult procedure, but when every aspect of the process was broken down step by step there was so much to remember.

Rikki and Dr. Scharf used their hips to push through the swinging doors of the delivery room, holding their sterile hands high to avoid contamination.

The woman was progressing rapidly. Labor tends to be much quicker for women, like this one, who have given birth before.

"This will be her fourth child," Dr. Scharf said, positioning Rikki at the foot of the table and showing her how to feel inside for the baby's head. "I bet this one will be a girl."

In the background was the amplified staccato of the unborn baby's heart, which still was being monitored constantly. With each contraction the *tap-tap-tap* sound would slow and then speed up again when the woman relaxed.

"Push! Push! Push!" the nurse shouted at the woman, who was struggling, her face wet with sweat and tears from the pain.

Then the black crown of the baby's head began to appear in the expanding vagina of the woman. Rikki got ready, holding her gloved hands near the emerging head. It was 2:06.

This final stage of the birth process goes very fast. Suddenly the baby's head, craddled in Rikki's hands, was out. With eyes squeezed tightly shut, the face looked like that of a cranky little old man not at all happy about entering this cold, sterile world.

But Rikki didn't notice this. She was too intent on easing the baby out, concerned that the protective vernix, a waxy substance that covers the newborn, would make the baby too slippery to hold. But everything progressed smoothly until the shoulders got caught. Rikki had turned the baby as she had been told, but now the baby was stuck.

Before she could say anything, Dr. Scharf was at her side. Rikki made room and the young doctor gently turned the infant in a special way. The shoulders seemed to pop out.

He stepped back and Rikki finished the delivery. Everyone was so intent on the drama of birth that it was a shock to suddenly hear the wail of a baby filling the room. It seemed so out of place. What in the world was a baby doing in this sterile, businesslike room where the adults were doing such serious things?

Rikki took the wailing baby in her arms.

And then, with almost equal suddenness, Rikki was laughing. It seemed incongruous, Rikki standing there, her green gown splattered with blood, holding a cranky-looking baby and laughing. No one had said anything. She just started laughing.

It was all over.

And she hadn't dropped the baby.

"It's a girl," Dr. Scharf called out, obviously happy at the accuracy of his prediction.

Rikki had been too preoccupied by the delivery to notice.

The nurse at the head of the table repeated this to the exhausted mother, who smiled.

Rikki carried the baby to the warming crib, gave it to a nurse, and came back to the delivery table.

"Oh, boy," she muttered to herself, not laughing anymore.

"You did real good," Dr. Scharf said.

"Oh, sure," Rikki grumbled.

It was 2:08, only two minutes after the baby's head had started coming out. It had seemed like an hour.

The C-section of the small woman went without incident. With Elaine assisting, Dr. James Connaughton cut through the lower abdomen, exposing a uterus swollen to the size of a basketball. Taking care not to cut too deeply, Dr. Connaughton sliced through the uterus and brought out a huge baby, almost twice the size of the one Rikki had just delivered.

"I bet she weighs over ten pounds," Dr. Connaughton said, looking at the baby being taken away by the nurse to the warming crib.

The baby had a slight cough. Aside from that she appeared fine, despite the earlier ominous sign of the meconium.

The pediatrician suctioned the mucus from the baby's nostrils and throat, listened to her heart, and put medicine in her eyes to guard against infection.

Then a nurse took her to the scales.

She weighed nine pounds four ounces.

□ □ □

C-section was common at Pennsylvania Hospital—about 15 percent of all births, or nearly three times the rate in suburban hospitals. One important reason for this, doctors said, was that Pennsylvania Hospital served a large poverty-stricken population.

Poverty was particularly cruel to the unborn. And extraordinary medical measures were required to help compensate.

Malnutrition, inadequate prenatal care, and ignorance accounted for many crises at birth. One in three babies born at Pennsylvania Hospital was premature, sick, deformed, or near death, according to Dr. Thomas R. Boggs, Jr., who was chief of the hospital's widely respected neonatology unit.

Sixteen of every 1,000 babies delivered at Pennsylvania Hospital died within twenty-eight days of birth. That was twice the rate of suburban hospitals and a little below the rate of 18 per 1,000 for Philadelphia. Big cities, being relatively poorer than the suburbs or the nation as a whole, had high rates of infant mortality.

Many of the mothers at Pennsylvania Hospital were teen-agers—so many, in fact, that the hospital had set up a special clinic for pregnant teenage girls. Some of the patients were thirteen or fourteen years old, with pelvises not yet fully developed.

One sixteen-year-old, who became pregnant a month after delivering her first child, asked to have her fallopian tubes tied off to prevent further pregnancies. The request was denied on the grounds that she was too young to make such an irreversible decision.

In the past, a large percentage of the obstetric emergencies at Pennsylvania Hospital were caused by botched illegal abortions. They were performed for women who lacked the resources to get a legal abortion by going through the farce of hiring a psychiatrist to swear that the pregnancy would endanger the mental well-being of the mother. These cases had become rare since the Supreme Court had made abortion legal.

Rikki had planned to go to dinner early. But that was before the obstetric emergency arrived.

At first it had seemed like a straightforward case. The pregnant woman was a twenty-five-year-old college student who already had a boy and a girl. Her pregnancy had gone to term, she had received complete prenatal care, and in all ways appeared healthy.

She was routinely admitted at 3:00 P.M. and taken to one of the labor cubicles. Initial examination indicated that her cervix was at six—that is, six centimeters across the opening.

Being a third pregnancy, the woman's labor was expected to proceed rapidly, which meant the cervix would dilate at a rate of about a centimeter an hour until fully open at ten centimeters.

But by 5:00 P.M. the woman was still at about six centimeters and in a lot of pain. She was in labor arrest.

Physical examination indicated that the cervix was becoming bruised and swollen from being pounded by the baby's head, which was being pushed by the birth contractions.

Concerned that a C-section might be necessary, the doctors had set the woman up in the delivery room. There was also concern because every time the woman had a contraction, the fetal heart rate, as indicated by the beeping monitor, would dip as low as 40 beats a minute—and then would take a long time returning to the normal fetal heart rate of 150.

Rikki sat on a stool close to the woman, holding her hand.

"They're getting you the pain medicine now," Rikki said to the woman, who had been pleading for relief. But most of the time Rikki said nothing. She just stroked the woman's hand.

The woman moaned from a contraction, and the fetal heart rate monitor responded by slowing, taking a disturbingly long time to return to normal.

A nurse came in with a tray of drugs and needles, and an intern prepared the syringe.

Rolling the woman on her side, the intern felt along her spine, found the right place for the shot, and then attempted to insert the needle. The woman moaned from the pressure. Rikki stroked her head. The intern could not find the right place.

Rikki was beginning to show the fatigue of being on duty for so long and enduring the stress of this woman being in such terrible pain.

"They're giving you the pain medicine now," Rikki whispered into her ear.

The intern tried two more times, eliciting groans from the woman, and then Dr. Robert Schreckengaust, the chief obstetrical resident, took over, deftly inserting the needle into the hump of the woman's spinal cord.

"The medicine should be working now," Rikki said.

"Yes," the woman said into her pillow.

"Good," Rikki replied, smiling for the first time in an hour.

The staccato of the amplified fetal heart slowed to about forty beats per minute and hung there for a long time as the doctors looked up compulsively at the device. It was an unfavorable sign.

Again the woman was examined. The cervix had not yet dilated. In fact, the opening seemed smaller, perhaps because of the swelling.

The possibility of a C-section was raised. The woman said nothing, but tears started to flow down the sides of her face, leaving glistening wakes across her cheeks.

They sat there for another twenty minutes, reluctant to do a C-section while there was still hope that the woman would start dilating. A senior physician came in, examined the woman, and said that she seemed larger than six centimeters and that they should wait for a vaginal delivery.

Rikki bent down to the young woman's ear. "He says you're doing okay," Rikki said. "He's a big honcho here and what he says is the way it is."

The woman stopped crying and attempted a smile.

The time dragged. No one said much of anything. Again, the only sound was the drum beat of the fetal monitor and the periodic moaning of the woman with each contraction. More and more often the monitor was showing heart rates below a hundred beats per minute.

This was disturbing to obstetricians because it meant the fetal heart wasn't distributing the blood with enough vigor. Most ominiously, it meant the baby's brain might not be getting an adequate supply of oxygen, which could lead to mild retardation, gross brain damage, or death.

Doctors were just beginning to understand the subtleties of oxygen deprivation in the fetus because only in recent years had the fetal monitor come into extensive use. In the past, the fetus was monitored only periodically—every eighteen minutes or so—with a fetal stethoscope, a method that could easily miss transient changes in the heart rate.

If there was truth to the suspicion that intermittent oxygen deprivation during the final stages of pregnancy was responsible for a lot of subsequent brain damage and retardation, then the benefits of monitoring should be seen in a few years when the babies delivered with monitoring reached an age when retardation could be fully detected.

The woman had another contraction, the heart rate dipped to forty, rose again but stayed below a hundred for a few minutes. Dr. Schreckengaust did not like this at all. The cervix still did not seem to be dilating, and the fetal heart rate wasn't recuperating adequately.

A C-section was needed immediately. The order was given and instantly a half-dozen people went into action.

A pediatrician was summoned to care for the baby the moment it came out. A nurse started swabbing the woman's abdomen with a brown disinfectant. Rikki, Dr. Schreckengaust, and the intern started scrubbing their hands at the sink. And the anesthetist was called.

The woman was sobbing now, knowing that there was no longer any hope that she could avoid this. They had her ready within minutes. Green surgical sheets had been draped around her abdomen, glistening from the still wet disinfectant.

Her arms had been spread out on either side and taped down to arm boards for the intravenous lines, giving her the appearance of being pinned to a crucifix. The anesthetist was ready at the head table with drugs and colored tanks of gases.

After waiting so long, the sudden rush of activity was startling. No longer did the staccato of the fetal monitor dominate the mood of the room.

Standing with her now sterile and gloved hands held high, Rikki looked down at the woman as the spinal anesthetic took effect.

"Oh, it's such a shame," Rikki said to someone standing next to her. "She'd been expecting to give birth and building up to it for so many hours. Now this happened. It's like waiting for a friend who never shows up. There's all sorts of anxiety and tension that's never released."

Moving remarkably quickly, Dr. Schreckengaust cut through the woman's abdomen and uterus and brought out a small baby girl. She was very blue but cried immediately, which was a good sign. Apparently no damage had been done.

Even with the spinal anesthetic the woman was crying with pain.

They hadn't given the mother gas immediately because it would have gone to the fetus through the mother's bloodstream, making the oxygen problem worse.

But with the baby out, Dr. Schreckengaust nodded to the anesthetist, who took the black mask and put it over the woman's tear-stained face.

Soon she was asleep. The only sounds in the delivery room were those made by the doctors quietly working over the woman and the shrill crying of the baby in the background.

□ □ □

It was after 8:00 by the time Rikki made it to the cafeteria, and all she could get was a cold sandwich, which she ate staring absentmindedly out at the now dark streets.

People carrying packages and flowers were coming into the hospital for the evening visiting hours, and the night staff of nurses and other hospital personnel were halfway through their shift. Rikki had been on duty now for thirteen hours and had another sixteen to go. Hopefully she would get a few hours' sleep, but such things are unpredictable.

The minute Rikki got back to the floor, Dr. Schreckengaust announced that a woman had been admitted with a possible ectopic pregnancy and they had to go downstairs to surgery to see about it. An eight-week embryo had started growing in one of the woman's fallopian tubes instead of attaching to the uterine wall and had to be removed surgically.

It was 10:00 P.M. by the time Rikki and Elaine got back to the obstetrics unit. It was decided that Elaine would cover until 2:00 A.M. and

Rikki would cover the remainder of the shift. So far it looked like it would be a quiet night. The sixteen-year-old had already delivered and there were no longer any women in labor.

Elaine sat down at the large bank of desks and started reviewing her obstetrical textbook while Rikki went off to the suite of on-call rooms and her bed.

Even though she was exhausted, it took her forty-five minutes to wind down and get to sleep. And even then it was a fitful rest. It was a strange bed, the room was cool, the blanket was thin, and in the back of her mind was the anticipation of being called out for a delivery.

All night long she dreamed of staring at a white wall. Then she heard a voice. And felt a hand shaking her shoulder. It was Elaine.

"Rikki," Elaine said, "It's six forty-five. We're supposed to go on rounds in fifteen minutes."

She had slept straight through. It was unusual for this to happen, but there hadn't been one delivery or admission during the night.

Rikki pulled herself together, her green scrub gown wrinkled from a full day of use, and made her way to the brightness of the physicians' lounge outside.

The day shift of doctors and students was streaming into the physicians' lounge now, slamming open and shut the steel lockers that held their books and white coats.

Talking and joking, they seemed so fresh and vigorous from the morning cold, while in comparison Rikki and Elaine, silent and cranky, looked wilted.

There was no time for breakfast so they went straight to the fourth floor and the start of rounds. The college student who underwent the C-section was already up in bed, talking happily on the phone, when Rikki came in to check on her condition. The other three women Elaine and Rikki helped deliver were also awake and in good spirits, watching the color televisions above their beds.

At morning report, which followed rounds, the cases from the day before were discussed, with most of the time spent on the labor arrest.

Morning report was conducted each morning by Dr. Edward E. Wallach, chief of the OB-GYN service, his staff sitting around a large table discussing the more difficult cases. Everyone agreed that the C-section was called for under the circumstances.

After morning report, Elaine and Rikki went to lectures. It wasn't until almost noon that they were ready to go home.

The bright sunny cold of the day felt good after spending almost thirty hours in the hospital, mostly in a room without windows, where day turned to night and back to day again without anyone's noticing.

For the rest of the month Rikki and Elaine would be on call every third night and in that time they'd each deliver another twenty-five babies or so.

In the future, when they looked back on the obstetrical rotation, the many births and nights would merge in their memories into one unclear event.

But the shift they had just completed would always stand out because it was the day they delivered their first babies.

29

The old man could not talk because the oxygen tube in his throat blocked the vocal cords. He could barely move because his wrists had been tied to the sides of the hospital bed to keep him from ripping out all the wires and tubes attached to his body.

The old man was angry and scared, and he wanted to get away from this place called the surgical intensive-care unit (SICU). It was obvious by the way his eyes opened wide with a mixture of outrage and terror whenever a doctor or nurse came near his bed, and by the way he tried vainly to pull free from his restraints and to kick people when they tucked his thin legs under the sheets.

"Don't be frightened, Mr. Gay," Matt Lotysh yelled, bending over the struggling old man. "I'm just going to disconnect this for a few minutes. We want to see how well you can breathe on your own."

Mr. Gay jerked his head away from Matt, trying to avoid the hands reaching out to the plastic tubing in his neck that connected him to the ventilator.

"You'll feel a lot more comfortable and be able to talk when we get this tube out," Matt said, easily overcoming Mr. Gay's resistance and disconnecting the tube. "But first we have to know that you can breathe on your own."

All the talking and reassurance meant little to the old man. He cared for none of it. He had spent too much time in the SICU. He had become paranoid, convinced that everyone wanted to hurt him.

All he wanted to do was get out of this place. It did not matter that he was too sick to live without the machines and the monitors and the people who kept bothering him.

□ □ □

The SICU at the HUP was quiet on this particular morning because it was Monday. Little surgery is done on weekends, and the patients scheduled for admission to the unit were still in the operating rooms on the floor below. They would not begin to arrive until about 11:00 A.M.

Three of the SICU's thirteen beds had been emptied in anticipation of the new patients, and three other patients would be discharged to other floors in the hospital later that day. Before the day was over all of the beds would be filled again.

Among those who would remain in the SICU were:

Jim MacMullan, fifty-five. An alcoholic, he was dying of cirrhosis of the liver after surgeons attempted to correct other problems caused by the disease. He was jaundiced and out of touch with his surroundings. Surgeons had suggested another operation to give him a little more time, but Mr. MacMullan's wife had refused. They had no more money, she said, and her husband would die in only a few weeks or months, at most, whatever the doctors did.

Harriet Anders, forty-nine. A week earlier she had been discharged from the SICU after partly recovering from surgery. She developed a post-surgical infection, though, and had to be brought back. The infection had spread to her blood and, apparently, to her brain. She was in a deep coma and the electrocardiograph showed only minor brain activity.

Harold Enrico, seventy-two. Shortly after undergoing major blood vessel surgery, he lost the ability to get oxygen into his blood because of a lung complication, and his kidneys stopped functioning. Statistically, his chances of surviving were less than 15 percent, but now, after six weeks in the SICU, it looked like he might make it.

Before the week was over, the thirteen-bed unit would handle thirty-three patients. Most of them would be discharged a day or two after they were admitted. Several, however, would spend more than a week in the unit. Four would die there.

□ □ □

The SICU was one of the three places in the hospital where a medical student could study the problems peculiar to intensive care. The hospital also had a medical intensive-care unit, for medical emergencies such as heart attacks, and a neurological intensive-care unit, for severe head injuries.

Students did not have to rotate through any of these units, and many preferred not to do so. Intensive care was a highly specialized form of medicine—one that most physicians would not need in their day to-day office practice—and it was often depressing and tense.

Some students, however, were stimulated by the tension and by the fact that their actions would produce an immediate and dramatic effect in the patient's condition. Such a student was Matt Lotysh.

"I like the acute situation," Matt said to a fellow student during a lunch break in the anesthesiology lunchroom. It was filled with dozens of doctors dressed, as he was, in the green scrub suits of the operating room.

"I like to know life immediately around me," he said. "I like to know it and feel it and touch it. I'm not aware of anything else when I'm here in this building. I like to be in control of my environment. In surgery and acute care medicine you have to be prepared for every situation. You have to know all the variables. Otherwise you will be caught short."

Matt experienced this total awareness when he was working with a difficult case in the SICU or assisting with open-heart surgery in the operating room.

□ □ □

Mr. Gay failed the breathing test and Matt had to put the old man back on the ventilator. He was still too weak to breathe on his own. Matt would test him the next day.

It was important to extubate a patient as quickly as possible—that is, remove the tube from his throat and get him off the ventilator. Not only did this make the patient feel better and enable him to talk but it also removed a potential source of infection and enabled the SICU to transfer the patient back to the ward.

The SICU could have a traumatic effect on patients. Many—like Mr. Gay—went temporarily insane if they lingered there. There was even a term for it—SICU psychosis. Patients already weakened by the stress of surgery began to break down like prisoners of war being brainwashed.

The SICU had few amenities. Everything was designed to provide the most intensive care possible. Ten of the thirteen beds were lined up in a huge room opposite an equally large nurses' station. The other three beds were in isolation rooms. For most of the patients there was little privacy.

The noise and activity were constant day and night. Telephones rang. Oxygen hissed. Electronic monitors beeped. There was the gurgle of someone's having his airway cleared with a suction device. Elsewhere there was the slapping sound of nurses pounding patients' chests to clear the lungs.

A crowd of people in surgical scrub suits and hoods rushed by, pushing a bed bearing an unconscious patient just out of the operating room. And always there was the light, glaring down from the ceiling, permitting no shadows to escape in.

The little high windows in the room were blocked by banks of monitors, which were constantly sounding alarms—usually because a wire had been pulled out of place, but sometimes because a patient was in distress.

Because the windows were blocked, patients lost touch with the world outside. There was no sense of time progressing. There was no day or night and the routine did not change substantially from morning to afternoon to night.

And always there was the reminder of the closeness of death, as patients in nearby beds died or came close to dying amid the noisy flurry of resuscitation attempts.

□ □ □

The first half of the week progressed smoothly. There were no crises or emotionally disturbing cases.

Five new patients were admitted to the SICU on Monday—four came from open-heart surgery and the fifth had a bad surgical wound that was becoming infected. Three patients were discharged and moved to other wards.

Five more patients were admitted on Tuesday. The four heart patients who came in on Monday were now strong enough to be moved elsewhere. The doctors were also able to discharge a man admitted the previous week after surgery for an abdominal aortic aneurysm, which is a rupture of the major blood vessel in the abdomen.

On Wednesday two more heart cases arrived, along with a man who had had brain surgery and a woman whose thymus had been removed. (The thymus is an organ that may play some role in fighting disease, but humans can live without it.) Again all of the heart patients from the day before were discharged.

About one-third of the patients coming to the SICU this week would be heart patients, which wasn't unusual. Persons who underwent open-heart surgery had a high risk of respiratory problems or heart disturbances during the first twenty-four hours after surgery, and they were taken immediately to the SICU instead of the recovery room. Only 10 percent of the other surgical patients required SICU care. Most surgical patients go straight from the recovery room to their own rooms.

The condition of the old-timers in the SICU—patients who had been there more than a couple of days—seemed to be largely unchanged.

Mrs. Anders was still in a deep coma, and no one expected her to come out of it. The blood infection had now destroyed one of her eyes, which under the circumstances seemed unimportant.

In the next bed, Mr. MacMullan continued to survive, though everyone expected that he would live only a few more days. His skin had turned a ghastly yellow from the jaundice, and he stared senselessly out of a skeleton of a head at the glaring panel of lights in the ceiling, bending his arms at the elbow, as though appealing for help.

Mr. Gay still could not be taken off the ventilator, but he was breathing for increasingly longer periods on his own before requiring assistance. He still hated everyone who came near him. He would yank his head back and forth, setting off the alarms in his ventilator, when the nurse shaved the white stubble from his face with an electric razor.

A high point of the week came when the doctors decided that Mr. Enrico could return to the surgical ward after six weeks in the SICU.

A handful of smiling, joking nurses gathered around the gray-haired man huddled in the wheelchair. He looked worried, clutching to his chest a hand-lettered calendar and two color snapshots of his son and a grandchild whom he had never seen because she was born while he was in the SICU.

Throughout his stay in the SICU, Mr. Enrico had kept the calendar and photographs taped to a stand in front of him as a reminder that time indeed was passing and that there were people to go home to. Now he was going to the two-patient rooms on the surgical floor, and he would be able to sleep in a dark quiet place.

But he was scared, as departing SICU patients frequently were. Having come so close to death, Mr. Enrico was preoccupied with his own mortality. He was no longer confident that his body was an autonomous, self-sufficient organism.

Instead he had become like a child, afraid to stray too far from the security of the SICU, his adopted home. Mr. Enrico did not want to leave the monitors and all the nurses and doctors. He depended upon them. He needed them to pull him back if his body failed him again and he started to slip away.

He tried to smile at his friends, the nurses who were urging him to come back and visit, but he was too worried about leaving. So he clutched the photographs and the calendar and did not look back as he was wheeled through the swinging doors.

□ □ □

Agatha Archer arrived on the floor late Thursday afternoon. She would die in only five days. But in that time she would have a more disturbing effect on the SICU staff than any other patient there at that time. She was assigned to Mr. Enrico's old bed.

It was not so difficult for the SICU staff to avoid emotional involvement with patients who arrived unconscious and died without waking up, especially if they were elderly and presumably had lived a full life.

But Mrs. Archer was a comparatively young woman in her early forties and until a couple of months earlier had been in perfect health. She was conscious when she arrived in the SICU, accompanied by her husband and two teen-age sons. They would be with her almost until the end.

It was hard on everyone to watch her decline, knowing that nothing could be done to stop the mysterious disease that was slowly destroying the organs in her body. Many in the SICU identified with Mrs. Archer; she was almost as young as they were and, until a few months ago, just as healthy.

Normally the SICU doctors tried to maintain a professional detachment from the patients. They felt this was essential to keep from being devastated every time a patient was lost—a more frequent event in the intensive-care units than anywhere else in the hospital.

Instead of dwelling on the ominous events surrounding death, they thought in sequences of problem-solving units, doing what had to be done at the moment. They were like pilots who were too busy trying to pull their planes out of dives to worry about the fact that the planes probably would crash regardless of what they did.

"It's a luxury you can't afford—spending your time and energies worrying about the things you can't do," Matt said to a friend during rounds. "It gets in the way of the things you can do. It interferes with my ability to do the job at hand."

Matt said he recognized the danger that a physician might become so detached that he no longer related to his patient as one human being to another. "This is something to which you must be constantly alert," Matt said, "and not allow yourself to slip over to the other side of the line and no longer care."

For the moment, Mrs. Archer needed drugs to dry her out because fluid was beginning to build up in her lungs, and some oxygen was needed to ease the burden of breathing. Everyone knew she would be dead within the week. But what she needed now were drugs and oxygen, and that is what they gave her.

Mrs. Archer's condition continued unchanged through Friday and for a while it looked as if the SICU would make it through the week without losing a patient.

Shortly before 9:00 P.M., however, John Kimberly was brought up. It was apparently a routine postoperative case, but shortly after he arrived his heart stopped.

Nurses, doctors, and students swarmed over his bed. Matt started injecting drugs ordered by the surgeon, who was pressing on the man's chest, externally massaging the heart to get it started. The heart would not respond. They applied electric paddles to shock the heart back to life, but this also failed.

About twenty-five people were crowded around Kimberly's bed as patients nearby looked with alarm at the commotion. The doctors would have to open him up again. Without taking the man from the bed, they cut into his chest and the surgeon started massaging Mr. Kimberly's heart in his hand.

A heart-lung machine was quickly brought up from an operating room on the floor below. For an hour the machine supported the unconscious man, oxygenating his blood and forcing it through his circulatory system. But the man's heart refused to take up the work on its own. It was no use. Shortly before midnight they shut off the machine and pronounced Mr. Kimberly dead.

It was a sad ending to a difficult five days.

The SICU had handled thirty-three patients since Monday, including an unusual number of terminally ill, chronic patients. Twenty-two of the SICU patients were discharged quickly, without incident. One died. Most of the remaining ten would do well.

But the prospects did not look good for Mrs. Archer, who had the mysterious disease, or Mrs. Anders, whose body was riddled with infection, or Mr. MacMullan, who was suffering from cirrhosis.

□ □ □

The development of the intensive-care unit has occurred in only the past twenty years. The units have substantially improved the care of seriously ill patients and undoubtedly saved many lives, but they have also created a number of social and ethical problems.

Because intensive-care units enable physicians to prolong the dying process by weeks and months at a tremendous emotional and financial cost, society has been forced to determine how much a human life is worth and when patients should be allowed to die.

Until the case of Karen Quinlan brought the matter into the open, physicians had been quietly and routinely answering these questions on a case-by-case basis. Rarely did they do anything as dramatic as pull the plug to a respirator keeping a patient alive, but that was only because they did not have to. Holding back fluids or drugs needed to maintain blood pressure or refusing to revive a stilled heart sped the doomed patient on his way just as effectively.

In response to the ethical dilemma, Massachusetts General Hospital, the main teaching hospital of Harvard Medical School, has developed a classification system that rates intensive-care patients from A to D. The D designation is given to patients who will no longer be given therapy because there is little hope that they can survive.

Difficult as it may be, allowing terminally ill persons to die sooner by withholding treatment has been an easier problem to resolve than the other major issue raised by medical technology—the economics of dying.

Should everything technologically possible be done to save human life? Is it reasonable to spend such large amounts of society's limited medical care funds to benefit so few? Is money no object when it comes to such things?

If the units were saving the lives of people who then went on to lead long and productive lives, then there would be little argument: Everything that could be done should be done.

The majority of intensive-care patients do return to productive lives. About 10 percent, however, are so seriously ill that it is obvious that they probably will not survive. What should be done for these patients?

The extent of the problem was demonstrated in a study by Dr. David J. Cullen, an anesthesiologist at Harvard Medical School, who for one year followed the fate of 226 patients classified as the least likely to survive.

Dr. Cullen's statistics were shocking. Fifty-four percent of the patients were dead at the end of one month. Seventy-three percent were dead at the end of the year. Only sixty-two patients were alive a year after being treated, and ten of these were in the hospital.

It had cost $3,232,647 to care for those 226 patients—more than $14,-500 a patient. If the United States attempted to provide comparable care to everyone near death, it would cost $28 billion a year, a figure equal to 69 percent of the total hospital bill of the nation, Dr. Cullen wrote in the *New England Journal of Medicine*.

Obviously no society is rich enough to make such an investment. Dr. Cullen felt that two things can be done to keep costs down—discontinuing intensive care as soon as it appears obvious that the patient will not survive, and keeping patients out of intensive care if there appears to be no hope.

The HUP has no formal classification system. But, said Dr. Harry Wollman, chief of Penn's anesthesiology department, which operated the unit, an attempt was made to limit admissions to the SICU to patients likely to achieve long-term benefits. It was not used merely as a place to put the dying, he said.

Hopelessly ill patients, such as Mrs. Anders and Mr. MacMullan, were allowed to remain only as long as the SICU beds were not needed for patients who had more than a fighting chance to survive. This process, however, created other problems, because the doctors did not always agree on who should stay and who should go.

If the doctors could not agree, an arbitrator was summoned. The arbitrator—a different senior physician every week—had the final word.

When called upon, the arbitrator came down to the SICU, looked at every patient, reviewed the medical records, and then decided who must make way for another patient. Arbitration was not an unusual event. Every week or so the arbitrator was seen walking through the unit from bed to bed in the process of making this difficult decision.

Mr. Gay passed the breathing test Monday morning, and Matt was finally able to take out the tube that had been helping the man breathe for a week.

The old man could not talk much at first because his throat was sore. But by that night he was grumbling at the nurses. By Tuesday, he was sitting up in a chair next to his bed, all bundled up in a blanket like a man on the deck of a cruise ship.

His eyes were still filled with rage. He was still psychotic, but he had stopped fighting with people.

Five of the other patients left from the week before were gone now— four had been routinely discharged and one had died. Like Mr. MacMullan, the dead man had cirrhosis of the liver.

That left only Mr. Gay, Mrs. Anders, Mr. MacMullan, and Mrs. Archer from the previous week. All the other patients in the SICU were new.

Everyone knew on Tuesday morning that Agatha Archer would not survive through the day.

No special note was made of her imminent death by the doctors on the anesthesiology team when they made their rounds. All they did was shake their heads when they saw that her blood pressure was falling despite the massive amounts of drugs they were giving her. The group then moved on to the next patient in the SICU.

This slight recognition, however, was more than they gave Mrs. Anders. They passed her bed without comment.

Asked about the difference, Dr. Peter Klineberg, the anesthesiologist on duty that week, said with some sadness:

"Mrs. Anders died last week. Mrs. Archer will die tonight."

It was an extraordinary statement, but Dr. Klineberg was unaware of its significance because he had been working in this strange world so long.

To an outsider, it was remarkable that the status of death could be assigned to one patient and scheduled for another, though by traditional social measurements both were still living people with indefinite futures.

In the afternoon the surgeons discussed the futility of the situation with Agatha Archer's husband, and it was agreed to discontinue further therapy. The blood-pressure drugs would no longer be increased, and a notation was made on her chart not to attempt resuscitation when her heart stopped.

The end came a few hours later. Her blood pressure dropped precipitously, she went into shock, her heart stopped, and she died.

Mrs. Archer's death was particularly hard on the nurses. Unlike physicians, who are forever leaving the SICU to attend lectures, view films in the x-ray room, or go to the laboratory, nurses had to remain at the patient's bedside. It was their job to help the patient's relatives adjust to the terrifying things that were happening, and it was difficult for them not to become emotionally involved.

It was this involvement with the patients and their families and the tension of trying to pull a patient through a life-threatening crisis that attracted people to this kind of nursing. Intensive-care nurses were competitive.

□ □ □

The problem of space became critical on Wednesday, and the arbitrator—this time, Dr. Wollman—was called in. He put on his long white coat, came up to the SICU, and went from bed to bed with Joan Richards, the head nurse.

Seven patients on the surgical schedule for the next day would need care in the SICU. Dr. Wollman had already canceled one of the elective operations because of the crowding, but three patients would have to be moved to make room for new arrivals.

Aware of the problem, the heart surgeon transferred Mrs. Anders to the surgical floor even though her condition was unchanged. Her brain function was minimal. Since she would die soon regardless of what was done, it would be better to let her die on a floor where there were ample beds than to keep someone out of the SICU who could benefit from the care.

Mr. Gay was strong enough to leave if he had to. Dr. Wollman told the surgeons of both patients that two beds were needed, so they obliged by "voluntarily" discharging their patients. They had no choice; Dr. Wollman would have ordered the patients moved had the physicians refused.

So on Wednesday, eleven days after he had entered the SICU, Mr. Gay was discharged. It was the fifth time in three months that the old man had left the SICU after being treated for one crisis after another in his lingering illness.

Mr. Gay seemed neither happy nor worried that he was leaving. He was just angry. He was also still psychotic.

□ □ □

A few days before finishing his four-week rotation, Matt attended a lecture by Dr. Klineberg on the stresses of being in the SICU, a subject of special interest to the Australian-born anesthesiologist, who was one of the three faculty members associated with the unit.

A half-dozen physicians and students were gathered around the table in the anesthesiology lounge. Dr. Klineberg was explaining what it was like to be a patient in the SICU when Matt broke in.

"It becomes your whole world," Matt said, staring down at the green tablecloth as though he could still see the intensive-care room he was taken to so many years ago after his appendix burst. "You lose all track of time. You lose all track of where you are. You just don't know if the room is on a cloud or in a cave. You don't have any contact with the outside. You just lie there all the time, drifting in and out of consciousness. As you stay in this state day after day, your sensory input becomes very bizarre. You start counting the cracks in the ceiling, imagining them moving, and you play little mind games to pass the time. That makes you psychotic."

Everyone was looking at Matt now, though he kept staring at the table, fingering the green cloth.

"I was getting a shot of morphine every three hours around the clock, but the pain would be gone for only about an hour and a half before it started up again. At the end of the second hour the pain was beginning to hurt really bad. But I couldn't get any more morphine because the three-hour cycle wasn't up. So I spent the last hour in agony.

"I wasn't scared. I just hurt. I hurt so bad that if I could have shot myself I would have done it. I definitely would have done it. Just to get away from the pain."

When Matt was finished, he looked up at the people around him and nodded, as though to confirm what he had just told them.

None of the doctors said anything. They remained silent for a moment as though out of respect for the personal things Matt had told them about himself.

Every doctor there had witnessed scenes like the one Matt had described. But Matt was the only person in the room who really knew what it was like to be a patient in a surgical intensive-care unit.

30

Theoretically the fourth and final year of medical school for the class of '78 began on September 5, 1977. But the day had no particular significance for the students.

Many of them weren't even in school that week but were traveling around the country, inspecting the internship training programs offered by various hospitals. After graduation they would go to one of the hospitals to continue the final phase of their lengthy education.

Those students who were on campus this particular day merely went about their normal activities, rotating through the various hospital services.

It was a sticky summer day, but beautiful just the same. The sun filtered through the trees along Hamilton Walk, casting jagged shadows on the pavement leading from the medical school to the hospital. It was reminiscent of the muggy day three years earlier when the class of '78 assembled at Penn for the first time and had a picnic lunch along the walk while upperclassmen told the new students what to expect in medical school.

Now the students in the class of '78 were the upperclassmen, and that first day seemed very remote.

The campus was peaceful. A couple of fourth-year students chatted for a while under the trees and then went into the college building to discuss internship programs with advisers. There was little activity in the student lunchroom. Outside in the hallway, a row of ugly steel lockers stood empty, waiting for the new first-year class to arrive.

Even though it would be nine months before the fourth-year students got their M.D.s, they had completed most of the required work for the degree. They now faced only one final hurdle to becoming physicians— getting into a good residency program.

These days, that was the only topic on their minds, and they were now visiting their favorite professors, asking for letters of recommendation.

Strong recommendations from nationally influential faculty members with friends in hospitals around the country greatly improved the chances of getting into good programs. And training in a good program would greatly enhance a young physician's career, or so the students thought.

It was an exciting time for the students. What happened during the next few months would determine where most of them would spend at least the next three years.

Some would return to their home states and a social life that had been disrupted by medical school. Others would be going to new places with better climates and more exciting scenery. And still others would stay in Philadelphia.

But this was also a stressful time for the students. They were in the process of being evaluated and ranked as prospective interns and residents. Their worth as professionals, and, some students feared, as people, was being determined by a committee.

This was the committee that assembled the all-important dean's letter, the single most important document in determining a student's future. Only two pages long, the letter told how the student performed in each of the courses taken at Penn.

Most important was the last paragraph—only two or three typed lines. It described the student as a "satisfactory," "good," "very good," "excellent," or "outstanding" candidate for a residency.

The evaluation committee spent hours determining which of these descriptive words would be applied. It seemed disproportionate, for what could a single word mean? But it was very serious business.

□ □ □

Upstairs in the medical college building, the five members of the dean's letter committee were finishing the process of evaluating the students in the class of '78, assigning to each the appropriate descriptive word or phrase.

The committee had been at this for the past two months. By the time the day was over, three of its members would have evaluated every student in the class of '78. The other two present this day were a surgeon and pathologist, since only students interested in these two specialties were being discussed.

"This student is described as being quiet and hard to evaluate," Dr. George E. Ruff, associate dean for medical student programs, said to the four other committee members sitting at a seminar table with him in the windowless room.

"I don't think we should include that in the letter. I don't consider quietness as a negative value."

The four other heads in the room nodded and Carol MacLaren, the assistant dean for student affairs, made a note to delete the offending phrase from the draft copy of the student's letter.

"I put him down as good," said Dr. Edward F. Foulks, a psychiatrist like Dr. Ruff.

The other heads nodded and again Mrs. MacLaren made a notation.

A pile of first-draft letters in blue folders filled with supporting documents and a photograph of each student lay on the table between Mrs. MacLaren and Dr. Ruff, the committee's chairman.

Mrs. MacLaren had written the first drafts herself, distilling the faculty evaluations already on file for each course into two or three sentences.

For instance, in describing a student's performance in a course on neonatology (care of newborn infants), Mrs. MacLaren wrote:

"His knowledge of the subject, clinical competence, and professional conduct were excellent. He willingly put in extra time, often staying up all night. He was described as an open-minded, hard-working student who showed unusually good judgment and adapted quickly to new situations."

The same student's performance in other courses was described with comparable enthusiasm. The last paragraph of the letter read: "We recommend him to you as a very good to excellent house officer candidate with excellent potential for a career in academic medicine."

The letters written by Mrs. MacLaren had been reviewed by the committee members individually the night before. All that remained to be done was to determine the final classification and remove particularly damning phraseology.

A letter about another student said that he had taken a five-month leave of absence because of depressive illness. The phrase "depressive illness" was deleted because the student's problem was not chronic.

Another student was described as doing well "in spite of personal and financial difficulties" that made it difficult for him to support his family.

" 'Personal difficulties' sounds psychiatric," said Dr. Foulks. The heads nodded and the phrase was taken out.

One member of the committee thought that a student should be rated "very good" while three others thought "good" was as far as they would like to go. They decided to rate her as "good plus," with the intention of reviewing her status when she completed her final courses.

The records of another student indicated that he had trouble relating to patients. It was fortunate, his professors agreed, that he was interested in pathology, where patient contact is minimal. The internal medicine faculty said that the student was not sure of himself. The surgeons said he needed more clinical experience. The pediatricians thought he was only satisfactory. The committee classified him as "satisfactory," the lowest rating given.

It took about two hours to choose the right word for each of the twenty-five students slated for evaluation this day. And even then the process was not complete. Students would be shown the letters and given a chance to challenge the evaluations before the letters were sent to the hospitals.

Only about five students out of a class of 160 would challenge, because the dean's letter was only a reflection of the scholastic records already on file. The records were open and all through the three years the students had been checking them each month as they completed each course. Still, any dean's letter that was challenged was reviewed by the committee.

About 75 percent of the students were classified as "good" or "very good." Usually no more than five would get the highest of all ratings— "outstanding" or "one of the top students in the class." Such a classification almost guaranteed them any residency they wanted. About ten students would get only a "satisfactory" rating. But even they would get a hospital appointment because there were more openings than there were graduating medical students, though the gap was narrowing.

It was a seller's market for students seeking house staff positions, unlike getting into medical school, where it was a buyer's market, with only one out of three applicants making it.

Most of the students would get one of their three most preferred hospitals. The fine shading of classification in the dean's letter was important only for acceptance into the most competitive programs, such as those at Harvard's Massachusetts General Hospital or Johns Hopkins in Baltimore. Only 20 percent of the class would go after such difficult programs. For those students, though, the slight difference between "outstanding" and "excellent" could very well mean acceptance or rejection.

□ □ □

The reference work most often consulted by the class of '78 at the start of the fourth year was the "green book"—the *Directory of Accredited Residencies* put out by the Liaison Committee on Graduate Medical Education and published annually by the American Medical Association.

The directory listed 1,671 hospital postgrad programs in the United States, along with other information the student needed in making a decision about where to go.

The directory listed what specialty training programs were offered. It described the numbers of annual hospital admissions and outpatient visits so that the student could determine how much experience he or she would be likely to get. The busier the program, the more likely it was that the residency would offer a breadth of experience. And, finally, the directory listed the salaries offered by the hospitals, which ranged from $11,500 to $13,000.

The students used a variety of criteria in determining to which hospitals they would apply. The quality of the educational program offered usually was the most important one, but there were many others.

Geography and living style were important factors. Some students preferred an urban setting and hence applied to hospitals in the major cities, while others preferred a rural environment. Some students wanted to return to their hometown areas, while others wanted to escape from them.

An efficiently run hospital with a lot of support personnel to do the drudgery work was an attractive factor, as were good physical facilities with accommodations for sleeping in the hospital on on-call nights.

Salary was probably the least important consideration because in the long run a prestigious program would be far more valuable in advancing the student's career. The high-ranking hospitals took advantage of this fact by offering lower salaries than less prestigious institutions. Unimpressive community hospitals offered the highest salaries of all.

Seeking a residency is a costly and time-consuming process; students often travel all over the country, interviewing at ten to twenty hospitals.

Medical students consider a residency with much more thoroughness than the average person checks out a job. Hospital officials, of course, interview the students, but the students are encouraged to question the hospital officials closely.

They interview faculty members and heads of the department they want to join. They go to the wards and talk to other interns and residents to see whether the program matches its description. They tour the facilities and check out the city and try to decide whether they would be comfortable there.

□ □ □

As far as Matt Lotysh was concerned, the only important thing was to get into a good surgical program that would prepare him to become a heart surgeon. It was a long educational process, one of the longest in medicine.

The average residency lasts only three years. But Matt would have to complete a five-year residency in general surgery before he would be allowed even to touch the heart. He then would undergo several more years of training as a cardiovascular surgeon. He would be almost forty years old when he finally opened his own practice.

□ □ □

Rikki Lights wanted an OB-GYN residency, and it had to be in Philadelphia. Ron was being maintained fairly well now on the dialysis machine and his band was beginning to make a small name for itself.

For her to move out of the area would have been to destroy this hardwon advance. But it was also important to Rikki to get into a good training program, and Ron realized it, so he offered to move if she couldn't get into a satisfactory program in the area. Reluctantly Rikki added the names of hospitals in New York and Boston to the ones to which she would apply. Philadelphia hospitals would be on the top of her list, though.

Rikki was very sensitive to the way she would be treated in the hospital and city she went to because she was black and female.

"You know you are different from everyone else," Rikki said to a white male friend who had inquired about her concern about these things. "You know that people are going to react to you differently. As a professional you want to go to a place that will give you the maximum amount of ease. Sex and race permeate everything."

Rikki had spent most of her adult life going through culture shocks. First there was the shock of going from her economically poor and all-black hometown of Sea Island, South Carolina, to almost all-white and exclusive Bryn Mawr.

No sooner had she adjusted to this than she moved from the all-female college to the male-dominated world of medicine. And now she was facing another move.

□ □ □

Mark Reber wanted to become a pediatrician and, for family reasons, preferred to stay in Philadelphia. Until recently he thought he would take the best program he could get in Philadelphia so that he could stay close to his family. Now, though, as application time approached, he decided that limiting his choices to one city might compromise the quality of his postgraduate education.

He widened his search area to include New York, Baltimore, and Washington, which had good pediatric hospitals and were close enough to Philadelphia for frequent visits. But still he hoped to get into a good program in Philadelphia.

□ □ □

The Nestor family was split. Jim and his wife, Becky, had come to Philadelphia from California yearning to return West as soon as possible. But Becky had now become very attracted to Philadelphia, had got a good job in the personnel department at Children's Hospital and didn't want to leave. Jim still longed for the West, though he had come to like Philadelphia a lot also.

Many hours were spent discussing the split goals and it was finally decided to apply equally to both areas, giving California the edge by putting a California hospital at the top of the list. Jim had decided that he would look for an internal medicine residency rather than cardiology or epidemiology because it was much broader and would keep more options open to him.

□ □ □

Kate Treadway wanted to do her residency in internal medicine at the HUP, one of the most prestigious programs in the world. The only better one was the famous program at Harvard's Massachusetts General Hospital. None but the very best students in the country were accepted there. Almost as a lark, Kate put Mass General at the top of her list, never thinking that she might make it.

The natural environment was the primary consideration for Randy Wiest, so his list of prospective hospitals sounded like an outdoorsman's guide to the natural wonders. Randy applied to hospitals in Augusta, Maine; Halifax, Nova Scotia; Vancouver, British Columbia; Pueblo, Colorado, and Denver. Because it had a superior program in family medicine, he put Denver at the top of the list, even though it was a large city. If he got the residency, he would live outside the city near the mountains.

The process by which students and hospitals selected each other was a very precise one and operated on a national level. It was not just a matter of students' interviewing at hospitals, which then picked the students they wanted. It was much more competitive and coordinated than that. The students would rank the hospitals they wanted to go to and send the list of hospitals in order of preference to the National Intern and Resident Matching Program in Evanston, Illinois. The hospitals would do likewise, listing the names of the applying students in order of desirability.

The process involved about fifteen thousand students in the United States and abroad and better than sixteen hundred hospital training programs. A rented computer in Chicago would match students and hospitals in order of mutual preference.

The results of the match would be announced at precisely noon (Eastern Standard Time) on "Match Day," which was March 15. Both the hospitals and the students were honor bound to accept the results of the match. The reasons for announcing the results nationally at a coordinated time was to give all students who failed to match an equal chance to call around the country to hospitals that might still have openings.

It was understandable then that the focus for all fourth-year students at Penn and elsewhere was March 15. That was the time when they would find out where they would go for the next and final stage of their education. But until Match Day, the students in the class of '78 had no idea where they would be spending the next three or more years of their lives.

31

It was obvious to everyone who came near him that morning that Dr. James E. Nixon was angry.

Dressed in a green surgical scrub suit, Dr. Nixon stood in the hallway outside the operating rooms, angrily puffing on his pipe and yelling to no one in particular about the incompetence of nurses, bureaucratic bungling, the plight of modern man in a world of technological excess, and the ineptitude of everyone but James E. Nixon.

It was well past noon, the time Dr. Nixon was supposed to have started an operation, and they could not find the patient.

Dr. Nixon ignored the surgical nurse at a nearby desk who was calling down to the floor to find out what had happened, and he roared at an innocent bystander, who rushed away:

"What's the matter with the cotton-pickin' people in this rinky-dinky place?"

"The patient is still in her room," the nurse on the phone called over to Dr. Nixon. "She has a one-hundred-and-one-degree temperature. What do you want them to do?"

"I want them to take the temperature again—rectally," he snapped back without looking at the nurse.

Shrugging, the nurse relayed the order and hung up the phone.

The operation would have to be canceled if the woman did have a fever, but Dr. Nixon didn't believe it for a minute.

Relighting his pipe for the tenth time in as many minutes, Dr. Nixon delivered a five-minute impromptu lecture on the quality of medicine in the United States and then yelled over to the nurse at the desk.

"Where's my temperature?" he demanded. "What's the matter—can't they find out where to put the thermometer?"

Giving Dr. Nixon a dirty look, the nurse dialed the phone.

Dr. Nixon relighted his pipe.

"It's ninety-nine point two rectally," the nurse called over.

Dr. Nixon puffed three times, pleased that once again he had uncovered incompetence and triumphed over it. The rectal temperature, which is more accurate than oral, was normal.

"Ask them why she's hot only at one end," Dr. Nixon said, leaving to get ready for the operation that could now be done.

Role models serve an important function in the education of a medical student. They demonstrate in very human terms the different things a physician can be. Many students will attempt to emulate the styles of the physicians they admire. But at a prestigious school like the University of Pennsylvania most of the doctors came from the same academic mold, so there are few styles to choose from.

The "Penn Physician" tends to speak with cautious and highly verbalized reserve, dress conservatively, and treat academic medicine with humorless and unswerving respect.

The unusual student—the one who stands apart from the crowd—would find Penn a lonely place if it were not for physicians like the loquacious and outrageous Dr. Nixon, head of the orthopedic department, chairman of the medical board at Graduate Hospital and former team physician for the Eagles football team.

James Nestor didn't realize that he would meet a character like Dr. Nixon when he signed up for the orthopedic rotation at Graduate Hospital. He had heard only that it was a good program, and he was interested in learning more about bones even though he had no intention of picking orthopedics as a specialty.

The pressure was off the students in the class of '78 now because all the grades and evaluations needed for the residency programs were in and the all-important dean's letter was on its way. Unless the student did outrageously badly and started failing everything, nothing that happened at school between this point and graduation in May would affect his career.

So students like Jim were beginning to elect courses that they were interested in or felt would fill a gap in their knowledge rather than picking the courses because they were required or would serve a tactical purpose for advancement.

Jim was pleased to discover the informality at Graduate Hospital, especially in the orthopedic department, after the pressured frenzy and one-upmanship at the HUP.

In many ways the orthopedic service resembled an Army MASH unit. Rarely did anyone take himself too seriously. And, if anyone ever dared, Ronald Nemetz, the chain-smoking former military medic and bone-cast man, would take him or her down a peg with a stone-faced, wry comment.

Instead of impressing one another with learned quotes from the *New England Journal of Medicine,* the "orthopods" would go about their business in the clinic and operating room, fixing up broken bones and chatting as they did like craftsmen in a workshop who were happy with their carpentry.

This was an atmosphere that Jim liked. He felt at home with orthopedics because it involved such engineering concepts as compression forces, torques, and stress factors.

He had expected to spend most of his time during the orthopedic rotation in the clinic, learning the mundane business of splinting and setting simple fractures and taping sprained ankles—the type of work the family practitioner in a small ommunity might have.

But soon he became engro   m the complexities of orthopedic surgery and started spending increasingly more time in the operating room, assisting Dr. Nixon and the friendly, easygoing Dr. Lee Osterman, who was senior resident.

Jim was fascinated with the way they could cut away diseased bone and fit in artificial parts to do the work the bone used to. Deformed knees, hips, and other joints of patients crippled by arthritis were being replaced routinely with plastic and stainless-steel devices selected from an ample supply of artificial human parts—the biomedical equivalent of a Midas Muffler shop.

Jim discovered that the orthopod's operating room was like no other in surgery. Other surgeons, who worked with soft tissue, needed only scalpel and needle to make their repairs. But the hard bone confronting the orthopod required tools of the workshop.

Hammers, chisels, and saws in a bewildering variety of shapes and sizes surround the orthopedic operating table. And instead of the hushed quiet of the conventional operating room, the jarring noise of buzz saws cutting bone or the metallic banging of hammers against chisels fills the orthopod's workroom.

The alarm buzzer on the electrical device in the operating room went off, but Dr. Nixon didn't look up from the unconscious patient he was working on. He was trying to nail a complicated leg brace into place, and it was up to someone else to check out the alarm.

The nurse jiggled the alarm switch and it was quiet for a moment. More often than not, monitor alarms sounded when the equipment or the patient was jarred, and no one got very excited.

But this time the alarm sounded a second time.

The nurse again snapped it off and on, and quiet was restored. Dr. Nixon didn't look up this time either, but a frown wrinkled his forehead above the green surgical mask that covered the bottom half of his face.

Once again the alarm went off, but this time Dr. Nixon jerked his head up, glowered at the nurse who was about to hit the switch again and bellowed:

"Would you stop shutting that cotton-pickin' thing off and find out what's wrong? What do you think you can do, put out fires by shutting off the fire alarms?"

Shocked by the rebuke, the flustered nurse searched through the drapes covering the patient and discovered that the ground wire had fallen loose. It was reattached, and momentary calm was restored to Dr. Nixon's operating room.

"Bring me your troubled masses," Dr. Nixon yelled at the ceiling as if to invoke the gods, "and I will make them nurses at Graduate Hospital."

The surgical masks made it impossible to see the expressions of the four nurses in the room, but the women were all looking at each other with eyes that seemed to say, "Nixon's at it again."

But Dr. Nixon didn't notice. Once again all his attention was on the brace. His anger and theatrics had come and gone so quickly that it was almost as though they had never happened.

The case in question was a difficult one. The woman was a severely malnourished thirty-eight-year-old alcoholic who had broken both legs, pelvis, and back in an automobile accident. The malnourishment and infection had complicated the healing process in the more extensively damaged of the two legs, and surgeons in another hospital had decided to amputate it. Concerned relatives, however, brought the woman to Dr. Nixon, who felt he could save the limb by using skin flaps from the other leg. But the procedure would require up to fifteen different operations.

This operation—the fourth in the series—took only about an hour. Dr. Nixon left, and the other people on the team paused for a cup of coffee in the lounge near the operating rooms.

"His bark is worse than his bite," Vicki Gast said to a newcomer to Dr. Nixon's operating room as she stirred her coffee. "You learn to love him after a while. You really do. But he does scare some people."

Mrs. Gast, the assistant clinical coordinator of the operating rooms, had the greatest respect for Dr. Nixon. Like Ron Nemetz, Lee Osterman, and other close associates, Mrs. Gast felt that Dr. Nixon was a brilliant surgeon if, perhaps, somewhat unusual in his personal dealings with people.

Mrs. Gast had begun working with Dr. Nixon almost five years earlier. She remembered the day well. The operating room nurses were holding an impromptu meeting to decide whether to refuse to work for Dr. Nixon because of his treatment of nurses. Just then a new nurse came bursting out of the operating room in tears, followed by Dr. Nixon, who pointed a finger at Mrs. Gast and yelled: "You're next."

In she went to assist in the surgery, and she has been at Dr. Nixon's side ever since.

Dr. Nixon was one of the few people who got in and out of Graduate Hospital without an identification badge. He refused to wear one on the grounds that it was dehumanizing to the hospital and the people the hospital served. "I don't feel you improve mankind by beating him over the head," he was known to say. "I can appreciate the administrator not wanting to have his typewriter stolen, but I don't want to turn my hospital into a concentration camp. The root word for the word *hospital* is *hospitality*. It's a hell of a thing when you post an armed guard at the door."

Dr. Nixon was also the only surgeon who didn't keep a lock on his locker in the surgical dressing room. "It's against my principles," he would say by way of explanation. "I refuse to associate with anyone who would steal from me." He had never lost anything because of his trust, but he did have to put a name plaque on the locker. Because it was the only one without a lock, every student or visitor would take it over—sometimes shutting out the trusting Dr. Nixon with their own locks.

With the exception of talking to patients and taking histories, most of Jim's time on the orthopedic rotation was spent observing. He did not get much opportunity to participate in direct patient care because the work was too specialized. In the operating room he did little more than hold retractors. Bone setting and casting was too tricky a business to entrust to a student.

Jim saw a lot of alcoholics on the orthopedic rotation. Many of the broken bones repaired by Graduate's orthopods resulted from accidents associated with drunkenness.

Jim took a history from one drunk who had fallen out of bed and broken his shoulder.

Another drunk had fallen down the stairs in front of his house and broken his neck. They had to keep him unconscious with drugs until the surgery could be done for fear that without alcohol he would go into delirium tremens (D.T.'s) and shake his head off the broken neck.

A football player was brought in after almost breaking his neck during blocking practice. Another young man arrived with two broken legs. He had been hit by a car when he bent down in the middle of the street to pick up some matches.

A lot of Jim's time was spent at the head of the treatment table in the clinic, reassuring patients while Ron Nemetz was at the other end, causing agonizing pain as he manipulated broken legs before putting the casts on.

"It will be over in a minute," Jim said, bending down to the forty-year-old man who was grunting in pain as he lay on the treatment table. The man, a drunk, had broken his leg when he fell from a barstool. Ron was at the other end of the table pulling the broken pieces of the bone into place.

"Aghhh," the man groaned, arching his back as though he had been zapped with a jolt of electricity.

Ron's voice drifted up to him from the other end of the table. "Come on, partner, ease it down a bit. It's only going to take a second."

Jim touched his shoulder and nodded comfortingly.

Ron pulled the broken leg once more.

"Aghhh," the man grunted, arching his back again. He didn't utter one word of protest or fear.

Soon it was over, and Ron started covering the leg with wet plaster-imbedded bandages that would harden into a cast.

"It's all over," Jim said to the man, whose face was wet with perspiration.

The man ignored him.

□ □ □

Every Friday afternoon a lot of the orthopedic people would end the week with drinks at Chaucer's Tabard Inn, a colorful and noisy bar a block away from the hospital on Lombard Street.

Here they would laugh and joke and tell stories about the week's events, and invariably the legend of Dr. Nixon would grow. He, of course, never attended these bacchanals.

"It's good to know that there's room in medicine for someone like Nixon," Jim said, pouring a beer and watching some nurses playing the bowling machine. "He's not like the typical attendings you meet."

The red-bearded and balding former mechanical engineer didn't like the brittle competitivenes of the medicine practiced by the younger, more aggressive members of the HUP staff. He preferred the friendlier and smaller Pennsylvania Hospital and he liked Graduate's orthopedic department.

Though he had come to understand how the pressures of long hours of work and crowds of patients could harden a physician, he still had no sympathy for doctors who treated patients as annoyances, distractions that kept them from lectures and textbooks. He particularly disliked the ones who called patients SPOS, an acronym that stood for subhuman pieces of shit.

"I feel like punching people out who say that," Jim told his friends. "I think if you let yourself get to this point you've lost the game. I hope I never get to that point. Even if you have been up all night, if you ever get to that point I feel you have turned an important corner. I sympathize with interns, but my sympathy ends at that point."

Jim was continuing to be disappointed with the impersonal nature of a lot of the dealings he had had with residents and attending physicians.

"Doctors have an interesting way of clicking off," he said. "By that I mean they have a way of not getting involved with you on a personal level. It's the rare doctor who can be friendly to you after you have gone through a rotation. It's very typical to meet a staff guy on the elevator two weeks or a month after a rotation and he'll ignore you. Some of it may be that you didn't make an impression. But another part of it is that they have a protective mechanism of clicking off. I think it's part of the business. Dante said that indifference is the very worst sin, and it's probably true."

□ □ □

Jim learned a lot about bones and artificial joints and a different way to practice medicine during his rotation through orthopedics at Graduate Hospital.

But the one lesson he would never forget had nothing to do with bones but rather with Shakespeare.

Dr. Nixon was hurriedly finishing up an operation, bandaging a freshly repaired leg, when for some reason he had need for a pin.

"A pin! A pin! My kingdom for a pin!" he said to a surprised nurse as Jim held up the leg of the unconscious patient.

"A horse! A horse! My kingdom for a horse!" Jim said.

Dr. Nixon said nothing.

"King Richard," Jim said.

Still no reply from Dr. Nixon.

"King Richard the Second," Jim added, referring to the Shakespearean play.

Finally Dr. Nixon responded.

"The Third," he said firmly without looking up.

He was right, of course.

32

Ms. Redmann sat tense and upright in the hospital bed and stared with fixed eyes at the anesthesiologist and medical student who had come to talk.

In less than twelve hours the fifty-six-year-old woman would undergo surgery, and she was scared.

It wasn't the surgery itself—a simple gynecological operation—that frightened Ms. Redmann. It was the thought of being put to sleep with gas and drugs. Time and again she envisioned the black mask being pressed over her nose and mouth and the panic she would feel as her senses left her. Her thoughts were fearful and melodramatic.

She would lose all control of her being. Her body and her mind and her very life would be taken over by these doctors she hardly knew. She would be alone. In blackness. Helpless.

"We'll put an IV line in your hand so we can give you fluids and drugs, and attach monitors to your chest. . . ."

It was the voice of Steve Levine, who was doing a rotation through the anesthesiology service. He was trying to calm the scared woman, both from genuine concern and because it was part of his job. Anesthesiologists traditionally visit patients on the eve of surgery to relieve their anxiety, using a variety of subtle psychological tactics.

But none of it was working with Ms. Redmann.

"We'll be right there with you all the time, Ms. Redmann," Steve said, trying to counter the feeling of loneliness that often descends on surgical patients.

"You will breathe some oxygen through a mask and then you'll wake up in the recovery room in time for lunch. What do you want for lunch?"

This was another psychological ploy: Get the patient to think of a positive event after surgery so that she doesn't concentrate on the operation as if it might be the final event in her life. But Ms. Redmann ignored the query, so Steve asked her if she had any questions of her own. She shook her head.

They all sat quietly for a moment, and then Steve got up, touching the woman's shoulder.

"Okay, if you have no questions, we'll see you in the morning."

Ms. Redmann was still tense and afraid. She would not be an easy patient to anesthetize.

□ □ □

Some studies indicate that preoperative visits by anesthesiologists calm patients more than drugs do. When an anesthesiologist visits a patient on the eve of surgery, he will ask a series of medical questions, take a blood-pressure reading, and listen to the heart with a stethoscope.

There is a technical reason, of course: The anesthesiologist needs to know whether the patient is allergic to drugs or anesthetics. But the primary purpose of the visit is to establish a positive doctor-patient relationship through the power of suggestion. Patients have come to know that physicians ask certain kinds of questions and listen to hearts with stethoscopes, so to do such things is to establish oneself as a doctor.

□ □ □

Steve and the anethesiology resident he was assigned to, Dr. Roger Moore, did all these things with Ms. Redmann. And the moment she was wheeled into the operating room that morning, Steve bent over her upturned head and welcomed her the way he was supposed to, so that she could see his face and recognize him and realize she was not alone. But it didn't really work. She was still terrified of being put to sleep.

She didn't say much as Steve put in the intravenous (IV) line and attached the monitors, even though he and Dr. Moore were trying to make diverting conversation. Finally the time came to induce unconsciousness, and Steve brought the mask to her face. She tensed.

Dr. Moore waved Steve off.

"Hold the mask a few inches above her face because of her claustrophobia," Dr. Moore whispered. She wouldn't breathe as much of the oxygen coming out of the mask, but she would get enough to saturate her lungs.

Later the oxygen would be mixed with nitrous oxide, a mild anesthetic. First, though, she would be put to sleep with Sodium Pentothal, which Dr. Moore had started injecting into the IV line that led to the vein in the back of her hand. In less than a minute the drug started to take effect. Ms. Redmann's tense muscles relaxed and soon she was asleep.

Quickly Steve positioned the black mask over the woman's face and added the nitrous oxide, and Ms. Redmann's respiration started inflating and deflating the big black rubber bag attached to the face mask.

Throughout the operation, Steve's hand would be around the bag, ready to detect any changes in the rate or depth of the respiration. Such changes could indicate that Ms. Redmann was in trouble or regaining consciousness in the middle of surgery because the anesthesia was too light.

Contrary to popular opinion, a patient is not simply knocked out at the start of surgery and brought back to consciousness when it's all over. Instead, the anesthesiologist walks a thin line throughout the procedure, giving the patient just enough drugs to keep him unconscious without excessively depressing bodily functions like heart rate and respiration.

Since the patient is always close to consciousness, the anesthesiologist must be constantly alert for signs that he is coming out of it. It could be a terrifying, if not painful, experience for a patient to wake up in the middle of the operation.

As Steve and Dr. Moore administered the anesthetic, Ms. Redmann's legs were strapped into stirrups, the lower part of her body was draped, and the surgeon began the D & C (dilation and curettage).

Since it was such a minor procedure, Dr. Moore was relying on the Sodium Pentothal—a very safe but short-acting anesthetic, which lasts for only ten minutes—in combination with the milder nitrous oxide.

"She's getting light," Dr. Moore called out suddenly.

Steve jerked his head up. He had been watching the woman's face and was surprised to see her right hand flailing the air, as though pushing something away. Her brain was picking up pain signals, but she was too far from consciousness to realize it. The surgeons stopped the D & C.

"Take the mask off," Dr. Moore said, injecting some more Sodium Pentothal into the plastic tube leading to the woman's hand.

If Ms. Redmann regained full consciousness at that moment, she would be terrified to find over her face the mask she dreaded so much.

Quickly Steve took it off, but not for long, because the Sodium Pentothal started to take effect again. The woman became quiet. And the surgery was resumed.

The minutes passed and Steve stood alert, his hand around the breathing bag, looking for changes in the rate or depth of respiration that might indicate Ms. Redmann was regaining consciousness.

The operation was taking much longer than it normally would because the surgeon kept stopping to explain things to his own students. If Dr. Moore had known what was going to happen, he would have chosen a longer-acting anesthetic than Sodium Pentothal.

"She's light."

This time it was Steve who picked it up. Ms. Redmann had started breathing more deeply and rapidly, indicating that the anesthesia was wearing off again.

Dr. Moore injected more drugs into the plastic tube. Her breathing slowed to a more normal rate.

Twice more the woman became "light" and both times she was sent under again with drugs. The doctors would not give her more anesthetics until she showed signs of needing it for fear of overloading her system with the drugs.

Such overloading isn't particularly dangerous in itself, but it lengthens the time the patient must stay in the recovery room getting over the effects of the anesthetics.

Finally the surgeons indicated that they were through, and the anesthesiologists started reversing the effects of the drugs and nitrous oxide by giving Ms. Redmann oxygen.

"Ms. Redmann! Ms. Redmann!" Steve yelled, bending down to her ear. "It's all over. The operation is finished and everything went fine."

Ms. Redmann groaned.

Anesthesiologists try to wake patients as quickly as possible because they are in danger when they're half-unconscious. The most frequent and lethal postoperative complications from anesthesia in strong patients are throwing up and suffocating on the tongue.

Because the anesthetics deaden the gagging reflex, a patient who throws up is in danger of inhaling the vomit and scarring his lungs with the stomach acids. And because the anesthetics also knock out the muscles that control the tongue, there's always a postoperative risk that the patient's tongue will flop back and close the airway.

"Ms. Redmann!" Steve yelled again. "It's all over and everything is . . ."

Suddenly she was struggling to sit up on the litter. Her arms swung out and she kicked at the people who came to restrain her.

"No! No! Don't get up!" Steve yelled.

She was grabbing at the nurse who was holding her, trying to get off the litter. It was a case of "emergence excitement." Sometimes patients, especially those who were afraid of anesthesia, will begin fighting to run away the moment they emerge from unconsciousness.

"Rest a bit," Steve said, holding Ms. Redmann's shoulders down. "There's no need to get up right now. Everything went fine. Just relax. It's all over."

The woman looked up at Steve with dazed suspicion.

Was it really all over?

□ □ □

In many ways the four years of medical school had been good to Steve. He had lost twenty pounds since coming to Penn and he looked trim and fit. Sharply defined features had replaced the soft, pudgy face he had in 1974.

Like many of his classmates, Steve, who was now thirty-three, felt that medical school had given him self-assurance and a sense of control, though it had not been a completely satisfying experience.

Steve and Laura, his wife, who shared with him the anxieties of the first autopsies and anatomy lessons so many months ago, were divorced now.

Sitting in the anesthesiologists' lounge between cases in his green scrub suit, Steve thought back over the four years of medical school.

"Yes, I've grown a lot in that time," he said. "The growth has come from the repeated exposures to the stress that a medical student has: giving case presentations to senior physicians; constantly being evaluated as a professional and a person; laying hands on patients; childbirths and successful codes (resuscitation alarms); short-tempered interns, hostile patients, good patients; fatigue; early-morning calls; the different cities I've been in; the different hospitals."

The educational experience itself had been disappointing in some ways. Many of the Penn students had criticized academic medicine as impersonal and excessively competitive and for stressing technology and science almost to the exclusion of human concerns. They said this even though most of them thought Penn was one of the most humane schools in the United States.

"Medicine is a lot of late nights and early mornings, bad tempers and hard work," Steve said. "In many ways it is intellectually a lot easier than it's cracked up to be. It's also a lot more routine.

"The academic medical world is a lot more cutthroat than I expected. . . . The world of medicine is not as attractive as I had envisioned. . . . I'm disappointed with the kind of people, the attitudes, the working conditions, the social milieu within which it operates."

□ □ □

The complaints about the impersonal nature of the medical education process were no surprise to the people who were responsible for that process. They saw the problem as unavoidable.

In a very short period, the students had to master an imposing mountain of material and learn what was virtually another language. Much of the training was time-consuming, conducted through apprenticeships. There was little time left for more human concerns.

Medical knowledge was so complex and diverse that the students had to move quickly from one specialized program to another, from on specialist to another, never having time to develop a sense of rapport with people or concepts.

The huge army of professionals required to provide care in a university hospital accounted for the impersonal nature of the environment, Dean Stemmler said. "I don't think you can avoid this. It might very well be the nature of the system. I don't think that it means the care is impersonal. It's the student's interpretation of where she or he is at in the whole array of students, fellows, residents, and specialty consultants.

"All you have to do to please students—and I wish we could do it all the time—is recognize them as being welcome and draw them to your bosom. Do this and they will love you forever. The funny thing is that when this very same student who is so unhappy becomes a resident and part of everything that is going on, he will think that this is the greatest place in the world. And some of them will behave to the students under them just as the residents they don't like are behaving to them now."

33

There was something about the patient that didn't seem right. Maybe it was the extensive way she described her symptoms. Or the slightly belligerent way she related to the doctors in the hospital. Or maybe it was the problem itself—low back pain—and the fact that she had been in an automobile accident.

Barbara Turner was not happy when the case was assigned to her.

Low back pain is a difficult medical problem to diagnose, and more often than not it is as frustrating to the student and physician as it is painful to the patient because nothing definitive can be done.

Bobbi, who was finishing up a four-week rotation on the neurology service at Pennsylvania Hospital, accepted the assignment without comment.

That's the way it is in medical school, she thought as she trudged off to the patient's room. A lot of boring and tedious cases are mixed in with the interesting ones.

Bobbi might have been more eager had she known what she was beginning. This was to be one of the most mysterious cases she would have all month. It would also reflect a problem that plagued women medical students in subtle and unpredictable ways: sexism, an unavoidable part of the hitherto male-oriented world of medicine.

□ □ □

Bobbi was counting the days until she completed this rotation because it would be her last one. The neurology course would mark the end of medical school. She would have nothing more to do but wait for Match Day. And two months later she would get her medical degree. From then on, for the rest of her life, she would be Dr. Barbara Turner.

Bobbi anticipated June and the start of her internship, or residency as it was now called, with both excitement and fear.

After so many years of schooling—twenty-three years in all, from kindergarten through medical school—it would be good to be finally taking charge and making money, even though the pay would be only about $12,000 a year. Also, she looked forward to being an active part of a medical team, having responsibility instead of being just an observer who was more tolerated than welcomed.

But Bobbi was also apprehensive. The medical degree might make her a doctor officially, but she didn't really feel like one.

It was one thing to be a student and suggest what should be done to the patient, knowing that no action would be taken until someone who knew more agreed. It would be another thing to be a new first-year resident and suddenly start making decisions and implementing them, for better or worse, without talking to anyone beforehand.

"I'm just holding my breath for the internship to be over," Bobbi said to a fellow student over lunch one day. "It's going to be a grueling year. You're low man on the totem pole. It's really going to be a shock to be telling patients in the hospital that you're the doctor instead of saying that the doctor is that guy over there. Now you're going to be the person where the buck stops."

□ □ □

Judith Lisa Byerly was wearing a nightgown and sitting in the chair next to the foot of her bed when Bobbi arrived with a male second-year student who was just observing. Mrs. Byerly was a severe woman who prided herself on being a good person who followed a strict moral code that clearly defined everyone's role in life.

Men were supposed to work hard and support their families. Working hard and being loyal were more important than having a meaningful relationship, a common phrase of modern society that Mrs. Byerly had come to despise.

Likewise the woman's role was clearly defined. And it was for the woman to raise the children, keep the house, and be loyal to and respectful of the man, whether she liked him or not. Mrs. Byerly did not like the women's liberation movement at all. In fact, she didn't much care for anything except following her rigid code and disapproving of everyone else who didn't.

Bobbi was wearing the medical student's short white jacket. A stethoscope poked out from her pocket. And her usually very sociable and friendly demeanor had been replaced by a businesslike, efficient, almost distant manner. Bobbi identified herself as a student doctor from the neurology service and said that she would take Mrs. Byerly's medical history.

A deep frown wrinkled Mrs. Byerly's forehead. She looked at this twenty-eight-year-old woman who had taken a seat next to her and felt that familiar surge of outrage building inside her again. Mrs. Byerly didn't see a student doctor, but rather an unusually attractive young woman with blonde hair and almost classic features who obviously was in violation of the code.

Bobbi asked Mrs. Byerly to tell her something about the problem that had brought her into the hospital. At that point Mrs. Byerly wanted to chastise this young woman, but she was, after all, a patient in a hospital who was intimidated by the surroundings and the people who wore white coats and seemed so in charge of everything.

"Well, look, I've already told this to the other doctors, but I'll tell it again to you also," Mrs. Byerly finally said.

Bobbi smiled a "thank you," and the woman started the long history, dwelling on the more dramatic aspects of the story.

"The first thing that you've got to realize is that I was a very healthy woman. I was never sick a day in my life. I walked to work every day and it was more than a mile. That's not bad for a woman over fifty, you know. Before the accident I used to be a saleslady in a department store. I was standing up all the time," she said.

"Accident?" Bobbi was looking at her firmly.

"Look," Mrs. Byerly said with annoyance, "let me tell you the story my way. I'll get to all that. I've got to do it my way because I've got all the facts straight in my head."

Bobbi's lips tensed slightly, but it was barely noticeable. She nodded, without smiling, for Mrs. Byerly to continue.

Mrs. Byerly continued to respond to the questions Bobbi asked, but when she did she spoke to the male second-year student who had accompanied Bobbi. It was a disturbing thing for her to do because the male student sat on the other side of the bed, and everytime Mrs. Byerly addressed him she had to turn away from Bobbi, who was the one asking the questions and was obviously five years older than her companion.

Mrs. Byerly rambled on about how active she used to be and how she always took care of herself. Finally she got to the automobile accident.

She had stopped at a light when a car struck her from behind. The impact threw her against the front of the car. It didn't knock her unconscious, but she couldn't get up because of the pain in her legs and back.

Mrs. Byerly said she had seen several doctors, had been to the hospital a couple of times and had received special treatments, but nothing would relieve the pain.

The case was remarkably similar to another one, involving a man, that Bobbi had seen a week earlier.

Bobbi asked Mrs. Byerly to get up and demonstrate how she could walk by going down the hall outside of her room.

Mrs. Byerly didn't like this at all and she demanded to know why she should do this. She had been humoring this girl long enough. It was enough that she had to do these things for the real doctor.

Bobbi bridled at the phrase "real doctor," but she remained cool and firmly explained why it was necessary, that her observations would be relayed to the senior physicians and would serve as the basis for discussing her case. Exasperated, Mrs. Byerly got up.

She walked down the hall with a stiff gait. Bobbi asked her to walk with her eyes closed while she stood nearby to catch her if she fell. Mrs. Byerly walked with her eyes closed, but she didn't fall.

Bobbi asked her to lie on the bed and then checked her reflexes with a little hammer and a tuning fork and needles to evaluate nerve pathways. It was a remarkable examination.

Mrs. Byerly seemed to tense slightly when Bobbi stuck the pins into her flesh below the waist, but she said she felt nothing.

She said she didn't feel the vibration of the tuning fork or the soft warm touch of Bobbi's hands or the prick of the needles—all different types of sensations that travel along different nerve pathways to the brain.

Her lack of feeling indicated that all sensation from the lower half of her body had been cut off.

Standing upright and walking is a surprisingly complex business. The brain must constantly analyze sensory data from the eyes and all the nerves that indicate the body's orientation to the ground. Instantly responding to this changing information, the brain maintains balance by altering posture and the position of the limbs.

Bobbi was dumbfounded. Mrs. Byerly was able to walk even with her eyes closed. How could she possibly maintain her balance if she had no sensory input from the lower part of her body or from her eyes?

Bobbi looked forward to the next day's rounds when she would present this case to the director of Pennsylvania Hospital's neurology department, Dr. Gunter R. Haase.

□ □ □

During their four years at Penn, the women students rarely encountered blatant sexism. All of them, however, could cite isolated instances like the case of Mrs. Byerly when they were treated in a condescending manner or at least not as equals to the male students.

Though all of the women wore the short white coat of the medical student, some people persisted in calling them nurses.

Vanessa Gamble, a black student, said one male patient thought she was a maid even after she had given him a medical examination.

Suzanne Landis said that a couple of times male physicians had even patted her on the head and back, so much to her annoyance that she complained.

Lois Garner told about a surgeon who always offered her the best viewing position at the operating table, giving her preference over all the male students. Katharine Treadway said she had had a similar experience in her surgery rotation.

The most blatant example of sexism anyone could remember was the now infamous lecture by a department chairman who kept making sexist references.

He didn't realize what he was doing, even though he was greeted with a roomful of boos every time he said something like, "This is the way to separate the men from the boys."

The sexism wasn't so severe that it seriously interferred with the education of the women students. But it was there on a very subtle level, just as it is in society as a whole.

Referring to one incident when a resident called all the male students in a group "doctor" and the one woman student "miss," Vanessa said:

"I think those attitudes are really insidious things. It might seem like a small thing. It's nothing obvious. Usually it's just a feeling. It's like a background. That's why it's not a small thing."

Nevertheless, blatant sexism was slowly disappearing from the white male-dominated world of medicine. So many women were entering medicine that they were no longer a novelty to be amused by.

Forty-eight of the 160 students in the original class of '78 were women. On a national level the percentage of women entering medical school doubled between 1969 and 1974.

In 1969, only 9.2 percent of the entering students were women. By the time the students in the class of '78 arrived in 1974, the figure had reached 19.7 percent. And in 1977 the number had gone to 25.6 percent. That is, 4,130 out of 16,136 first-year students were women.

□ □ □

Dr. Haase was one of the more distinctive role models for the students in the class of '78, almost the antithesis of the equally interesting Dr. Nixon. The fifty-three-year-old neurologist was a graduate of the University of Munich and spoke with a slight German accent, which added to his worldly and cultured air.

This dignified image was enhanced by his white wavy hair and horn-rimmed glasses, which covered only the lower half of his eyes.

He had the trim figure of a tennis player or skier (he was both), and he was forever mixing references to Wagnerian operas, current literature, or observations from his many travels around the world into his clinical dissertations.

Students would ask him what neurology offered as a specialty and why he himself had gone into it twenty-five years earlier. And Dr. Haase would explain it to them:

"My attraction to neurology was partly out of the need to know what makes people tick. Neurology has the appeal of a certain neatness of logic. You have to know a fair amount of anatomy and physiology and something about pathology. It permits quite orderly consequential thinking."

A large part of neurology consists of trying to locate the source of damage in the nervous system by doing such things as watching the types of seizures a patient has or comparing the strength and reflexes of one side of the body with those on the other.

"Neurologists like moving from the concrete to the abstract," Dr. Haase would say. "Watching the wiggle of the big toe may tell us something about what is happening far removed from it—something happening in the spinal column or even in the brain."

He conceded that neurology appeared to be a more depressing specialty than many. He estimated that neurologists could do nothing for 25 percent of the patients they saw, but he thought this was no worse than in most other specialties.

Neurology only appears to be grimmer, he would say, because neurologic disease so often strikes the brain and disrupts the most human of all qualities—thinking, relating, feeling.

"I think," Dr. Haase would say, fingering his horn-rimmed glasses, "that some persons, who are not ready to accept some of the grimness of life, oughtn't to have gone into medicine in the first place. The student who has a high emotional need to have everyone well and everyone happy probably would be best in obstetrics.

"I think a person who enters medicine ought to be able to tolerate a certain amount of the grimness of life . . . ought to be able to recognize that sometimes we can do nothing and life rolls on all the same."

And so it was that this sensitive, cultured man, with so much empathy for the incurably ill, was brought into the case of Judith Lisa Byerly.

□ □ □

Morning rounds began with Mrs. Byerly's case. The white-coated neurology team, including Dr. Haase, had gathered in a conference room down the hall from Mrs. Byerly's room, and Bobbi presented the case.

As she talked, providing fact after fact without comment, the inconsistencies were immediately obvious to everyone. Dr. Haase became increasingly uneasy.

Bobbi told how Mrs. Byerly could walk yet had no sensation below the waist. She told him about the automobile accident and, as an aside, about the lawsuit Mrs. Byerly had started.

"Is she incontinent?" Dr. Haase asked.

Bobbi said no. Dr. Haase frowned. People who are paralyzed below the waist almost always lose control of urination or defecation.

Bobbi told how Mrs. Byerly seemed to wince at the pin pricks but said she felt nothing. And she related how insistent the woman was on telling her story her own way.

"I better see her now," Dr. Haase said abruptly in the middle of Bobbi's presentation. "I feel I am developing too many attitudes toward her."

The team followed him and Bobbi down the hall. Dr. Haase made his way to Mrs. Byerly's room, introduced himself, and explained that he had come to examine her further.

Dr. Haase put Mrs. Byerly through many of the same tests Bobbi had already done. Although he was very friendly, his manner was much more authoritative and less leisurely than Bobbi's.

Mrs. Byerly continued to give excessively long descriptions of her complaint, but as she kept talking, Dr. Haase used the time to examine her, throwing questions in as he did.

It was not so easy for her to take over the interview from Dr. Haase, and soon Mrs. Byerly was saying "Yes, sir," and "No, sir" after every other question.

Rolling Mrs. Byerly face down and baring her midriff, Dr. Haase took a needle from the lapel of his long white coat (it's the trademark of neurologists—they all have pins in the lapels of their hospital jackets) and started sticking her.

"Tell me when you feel the needle, Mrs. Byerly," he said.

Repeatedly stabbing the woman, Dr. Haase worked the needle from the bottom of Mrs. Byerly's torso up past the waist. As soon as she said she could feel the prick, he stopped and started moving up another line with his needle, each time a bit farther to the left.

In this manner, he moved across Mrs. Byerly's body. Everytime Dr. Haase went above the navel, Mrs. Byerly called out.

"It seems to form a straight line across her back and front at this point," Dr. Haase said, looking up at the students and doctors gathered at the foot of the bed.

Mrs. Byerly seemed to feel every sensation above the imaginary line, but none below it.

Human neurology and Mrs. Byerly's sensation of pain didn't agree. Because of the way the nerves are hooked up—each set responsible for transmitting sensations from different levels along the torso—the imaginary line should have dipped at the crotch instead of going straight across.

Dr. Haase wiggled Mrs. Byerly's toes. She said she could feel nothing. He scraped a pointed stick along the instep of her foot. Involuntary reflexes caused the toes to curl.

When Dr. Haase told Mrs. Byerly to roll over in bed, she used her legs to help her in this maneuver. But when he asked her to draw her legs toward her chest, Mrs. Byerly said she could not move them at all.

Dr. Haase asked Mrs. Byerly a few more questions, made additional tests and then left with his team in tow. A few minutes later the team was sitting around a table, discussing the unusual case of Judith Lisa Byerly.

At first Dr. Haase seemed convinced that Mrs. Byerly was a malingerer.

"Her reflexes are perfectly intact," he said, musing over his findings, "yet Mrs. Byerly says she can't feel anything below the waist. Ask her questions and her answers only cloud the issue further. There are so many things with this woman that are inconsistent with medicine, or at least medicine as we know it."

But Dr. Haase didn't want to make a socially condemnatory diagnosis like malingering without first ruling out other possible explanations. To do otherwise, he felt, would be unfair to the patient.

Perhaps Mrs. Byerly was a hysteric who unknowingly feigned a paralysis rather than concede that age was weakening her body. Or maybe there was yet another psychiatric explanation.

No, Dr. Haase said, he would prefer to have a psychiatrist see her before making a firm diagnosis.

At this time all he was prepared to say was that Mrs. Byerly's apparent incapacity was limited only to those functions she had conscious control over. All involuntary functions—such as reflexes—were in fine working order.

Mrs. Byerly had been much more respectful to Dr. Haase than to Bobbi. A large part of that was because Dr. Haase was older and more in command. But another, more subtle reason, was that Bobbi was a woman.

Barbara Turner would never again encounter the subtle sexism of Mrs. Byerly.

Bobbi left for a five-week vacation in Europe shortly after her involvement in the case and never did find out how the matter was resolved.

On the recommendation of Dr. Haase, Mrs. Byerly's primary physician referred her to a psychiatrist for evaluation and possible therapy. From all the neurologists could tell, there was nothing wrong with her body.

□ □ □

Mrs. Byerly underwent intense one-on-one psychotherapy twice a week for several months. At first she resisted it and there was little improvement.

The automobile accident lawsuit was settled out of court for considerably less money than Mrs. Byerly had hoped for, but her lawyer advised her against pursuing the case further.

She stayed in therapy, however, and Mrs. Byerly started discussing fears she had about growing older and the fact that her marriage wasn't doing well at all.

She switched to group therapy, which included one other woman her age who was also having trouble adjusting to her advancing years.

Slowly Mrs. Byerly began to feel some sensation in her lower back and walking and moving about began to be easier for her. The physical impairment flared up now and then. She would tell her group about it, but always the other people seemed to find some emotional problem associated with the sudden relapses. This annoyed Mrs. Byerly, but she had to agree that on the average she was feeling better than she did before starting psychotherapy.

□ □ □

Though the sensitive Dr. Haase was a unique and excellent role model for many, he had one serious problem as far as a growing number of students were concerned: He was the wrong sex. Women students wanted female role models. And no matter how attractive an example a male physician might offer, not being a woman was a serious handicap.

When the class of '78 started at Penn, only 56 of the 1,001 physicians at the HUP were women. Women constituted only 2.4 percent of the hospital's 545 attendings, the senior physicians who set the tone. And they made up only 9.4 percent of the house staff, which consisted of the interns, residents, and fellows who worked most closely with the students.

Women students who were not prepared to give their entire lives over to medicine—sacrificing family, friends and outside interests—found the male doctors at the HUP particularly unsuitable as role models.

The prototype HUP attending spends from seven in the morning until nine at night in the hospital," said Deborah Spitz. "If he has children, he never sees them, and if he has a wife, I don't know when they see each other. I wouldn't call it much of a relationship. It's particularly hard for women because they have always been saddled with raising children or finding someone who will. I just don't find very many doctors looking for creative solutions to the problem."

Suzanne Landis became acutely aware of the lack of role models the moment she began her hospital rotations in the second year.

"When I started my clinical rotations," she said, "I realized that there just weren't any women. Then I said, 'Don't be so picky; just look for a man to model after.' " But it wasn't until Suzanne took rotations outside the Penn network of hospitals that she found a physician—a man—she could consider a suitable role model.

With the striking increase in the number of women entering medical school, the lack of suitable female role models would soon be remedied as those women now in the educational pipeline found their way into positions of authority.

In fact, the class of '78 was probably the last class at Penn to endure such a stark shortage of women doctors. Just as the class of '78 was starting its final year of training, the HUP's departments of medicine and OB-GYN appointed an unprecedented number of women house staff officers.

Ten of the twenty-one first-year residency openings in the medicine department and five of the six positions in obstetrics-gynecology went to women.

Reverse discrimination?

Not at all, said Dr. Luigi Mastrolanni Jr., OB-GYN chairman, and Dr. Laurence H. Beck, head of the medicine department's selection committee for residents at HUP. More women than ever before were applying, and those who applied last year were, on the average, better qualified than the men.

More than five hundred persons applied for the twenty-one openings in the medicine department. And even though only 30 percent of the applicants were women, almost 50 percent of the openings—ten of twenty-one—went to women. The years before, only three women made it. The success of women getting into OB-GYN was even more striking since only 30 percent of the two hundred obstetrics-gynecology applicants were women.

□ □ □

The large influx of women into medicine undoubtedly will change the style of medical care practiced in this country. But no one is sure just how.

It had been thought that women, being more strongly oriented by culture toward family and home, would flock to medical specialties with more regular hours such as radiology or pathology, or salaried positions such as those in emergency room medicine. But the sudden upsurge in the number of women going into such competitive and time-consuming programs as the medicine department's at the HUP put such a theory into question.

Dean Stemmler was reluctant to predict the changes.

"I think we are expecting that the women will moderate the harsh relationships that are attributed to male professionals in medicine," he said. "They are expected to bring a softening influence. But I don't know if that will be true. For one thing, I think that the women themselves are going to be influenced by the professional role of being a physician."

Katharine Treadway, one of the top students in the class, challenged the thought that women students tended to be softer than the men.

"Supposedly there are certain feminine characteristics that would be helpful in the physician's role," she said. "But I'm not so sure. In many ways it comes down to each individual, regardless of what sex, whether they are comfortable dealing with people. I think there are a lot of fellow male students who are intensely concerned with their patients' emotional well-being. They spend a lot of time dealing with the patient's fears.

"It's hard to think in stereotypes when you see the individuals."

34

A half-dozen men were standing on the street corner in the west Philadelphia ghetto and every one of them was looking at Rikki Lights.

Rikki was standing in the doorway of a storefront, yelling through the crack of the chained door.

"Hey" she yelled. "It's me, Rikki. Let me in." From inside the store came the electrified roar of the Gilliam Brothers band.

Rikki looked out of place in the ghetto. She was wearing the short white coat of a medical student and carrying a little black physician's bag.

"Hello in there," she yelled again, louder this time. "It's Rikki. Let me in."

Two teen-age youths standing on the corner started pointing at Rikki and laughing.

Suddenly the music stopped. Rikki yelled into the silence and soon the grinning face of a big man appeared in the doorway.

He opened the door wider, and Rikki, the medical student, walked into her other world—the world of black musicians, playwrights, poets, and artists.

□ □ □

Many black medical students say they must work harder than their white classmates because they have to contend with a subtle racism that exists in this predominantly white and male environment.

Significant numbers of blacks in medicine are a comparatively recent phenomenon. Even now, only about 2 percent of the physicians in private practices are black, though 12 percent of the United States population is black.

Only since 1969 have Penn and other medical schools started to deal with this imbalance. In more than two centuries—between 1765, when Penn's medical school began, and 1968—only thirty-six black physicians were graduated from Penn. Rikki's class had twenty-two black students, the largest number in the school's history.

The black students in the class of '78 were strong in their praise of Penn.

"If I had to pick a place in the country with the lowest amount of discrimination," said Ronald Cargill, "it would be here at the University of Pennsylvania."

"When I came here I was really looking for it [overt discrimination]," said Conrad Kirklyn King, Jr., "but then I stopped looking for it, because it wasn't here. If I was grading Penn on how they treated minority students, I'd have to give them an A."

Other blacks said they had run into minor problems on occasion, but they felt that Penn was the best school in the city, if not the nation, for blacks, considering what their friends at other medical schools had told them.

Despite this glowing praise, almost all of the students recalled minor incidents and more serious problems that grew out of the racism that had existed for so long. These problems occurred in the hospital as well as on the Penn campus.

Rikki complained about the lack of eye contact between a few white physicians and the black students. Many other blacks had the same complaint.

"I've had residents who would not look me in the eye, and that's a problem," Rikki said. "There's an intimacy of teaching in medicine. If the person who is teaching you has difficulty establishing personal contact, that directly affects your ability to learn." She said that the same residents apparently had no trouble looking her white classmates in the eye.

The problems are compounded for the handful of black students from Africa.

"When people first see me, they think I'm just a regular black student, but when I start speaking, they know there is something different about me," said Hagos Tekeste from Eritrea, northern Ethiopia, speaking with a clipped accent.

"You have to work harder to convince them that you know what you're talking about. They think because you speak with an accent that you don't know enough medicine."

□ □ □

One particularly annoying problem for black male students was being hassled by city police.

Ron Cargill, who favored a conspicuous mode of dress featuring stylish clothes and his famous broad-brimmed hats, wasn't the only black student to be stopped, though he held the record with fifteen encounters.

Andrew Henderson had been stopped twice by police, once on the Penn campus and once at Thomas Jefferson University Hospital on the other side of Philadelphia. He was coming out of Jefferson after visiting his wife, a medical student, who had just had a baby.

The officers handcuffed him, hit him a couple of times in the chest with nightsticks, and took him to the police station, where a witness to the robbery that they were investigating said he didn't look at all like the robber.

During the couple of years when he drove a luxury car, Andrew had been stopped by the police and had his identity checked eight times.

Victor Battles was stopped five times in his eight years at Penn. (He attended the school as an undergraduate.) On one occasion, he was stopped by the city police highway patrol for no apparent reason and was taken to the police station after the officers discovered that he owed six parking tickets.

On another occasion, he was questioned while he stood outside his house on the Penn campus. Apparently the police thought that he was a lookout for some illegal activity. They did not take him away.

"I humbled myself to keep anything bad from happening," Victor said.

Bruno Cole, another black student, was stopped and questioned on two occasions but was not abused. Once he asked the police why they were demanding identification, and they told him that it was a high-crime area and that they were checking people routinely.

□ □ □

Rikki seemed to take on a new personality the moment she entered the storefront rehearsal hall and the band started practicing again. She dropped her physician's bag on a nearby bed, stripped off her white coat and shoes, and began moving in time with the music.

Ron was perched behind a cluster of drums, sweating from the exertion of making music. He was too lost in the sound to acknowledge Rikki's smile.

The long dimly lit room was furnished with discarded furniture and other items that hadn't cost money. But it was comfortable, almost sensuous in its appearance.

A couple of beds with colorful throws and pillows for backrests were arranged in the front to encourage people to sit down and talk. Posters from record companies and draped fishnets hung on the walls.

Hammered onto the walls around the band were hundreds of egg cartons—makeshift acoustic tiles to keep the music from echoing. In the dim light they formed an attractive pattern, almost like an Oriental rug.

Still moving with the strong beat of the music, Rikki looked at the ceiling, lost in thought. She had just left Presbyterian Hospital, only a mile or so east of this place. But as far as Rikki was concerned, for the moment the hospital was all but forgotten.

Ron had been playing steadily for more than two hours after spending all morning tied to the machine. Doctors had discussed with him the possibility of trying another transplant, but Ron had been so disillusioned by the last tragic experience that he refused.

For better or worse he would remain married to the machine. The machine was keeping him alive, but some days were better than others. Frequently he felt tired and washed out and depressed.

Physicians were concerned that the fistula—the vein and artery that had been spliced for attachment to the machine—was weakening and might blow out like a weak inner tube. They wanted to put a new one in Ron's right arm, but he refused this also. He didn't want to use up another fistula site because once the few in the arms and legs were used up there would be no way to attach him to the machine.

The band was playing "Ethiopia," a haunting melody written by Ron shortly after his transplant failed. The piece had a slightly Oriental quality, probably because of the soprano sax. Time and again the clear, pure sound of the sax would enunciate the theme of "Ethiopia" while the other instruments played with it—running away from it but always coming back.

Rikki had become a member of the fledgling band, which was beginning to get good bookings. She didn't play an instrument, but read her vibrant poetry instead, sometimes alone and sometimes with her husband's band playing behind her. It was a strange but appealing combination.

After a time, the band stopped and the members joked back and forth as they got ready to leave. Rikki wanted them to play "Ethiopia" again, but the man on the synthesizer, Randy, from Swarthmore College, didn't want to play anymore. He was broke and hungry and didn't feel like it, he said.

Rikki bribed him with a dollar for a Gino's hamburger, so Randy and the other players went back to their instruments. The other musicians didn't need a bribe. Ron was smiling as he picked up the beat with his drums. And once again Rikki was lost in the music, her gyrating body throwing dancing shadows on the wall.

□ □ □

For most of the black students the shock of moving back and forth between the black and white cultures was not particularly traumatic, mainly because they had been doing it for so long.

Virtually all of the American black students had spent many years in predominantly white high schools and undergraduate colleges to get to medical school. They had long since acclimatized to the white world and learned to live in it.

It wasn't like snatching a black off of a ghetto street corner, where he had spent his life in semiliterate persuits, and plunging him into the intellectually demanding world of medicine.

Many of the black students came from middle-class black families with many of the middle-class standards and expectations. If anything, medical school merely continued a process that had been going on for years.

Many black leaders have hoped that more black doctors would help improve the care of black ghetto patients because black doctors would supposedly bring a higher level of concern for their people to their profession.

Also the inclusion of people from varied economic, social, and racial backgrounds supposedly would make the medical profession richer and more diverse, just as women should bring something special to it. But working for years in white-dominated educational and professional systems conceivably could make blacks less concerned about their own race. None of the blacks in the class of '78 thought this would happen to them.

"The system is going to change me," Rich Ellison said. "It changes us all. But I would like to think that the system is not going to rob me of my basic sense of identity. In order to get through the system, we, as blacks, have got to make certain adjustments, but I don't think this will weaken the blacks' effect on medicine. Just the fact that there are more blacks in the system will change medicine. It will be a significant change."

□ □ □

The majority of blacks didn't think the medical environment significantly altered their behavior, not any more than it did the white students'. But that was because the middle-class blacks and whites were already very similar in customs and behavior. For an extraordinary student like Rikki, however, most environments would feel confining, let alone the proper and restricted medical profession.

She felt suffocated by the white world of medicine, where the bywords were conservative dress, conservative talk, and conservative thinking.

She wore a turban while working in the emergency room and a nurse told her, "You don't wear rags like that on your head in here."

"In the hospital I can't laugh like I want to," Rikki would complain to Ron when she got home. "I can't talk like I want to. I cannot come close to people like I want to. 'Unprofessional' is the label they put on you. They would say you are wild. I have big gestures, but in medicine you can't have big gestures," Rikki said, flinging out her hands for emphasis, inadvertently demonstrating her point. "You have to learn how to distance yourself from people, and I think that the medical people have gone too far."

Her successes in the world of art annoyed some of her medical colleagues, just as the lack of art and creativity in medicine depressed her. Some interns and residents were antagonistic toward her and thought interest in anything but medicine was sinful.

She got a poor evaluation in her obstetrics course from a resident who thought she didn't show enough interest in her work, that she seemed to prefer her writing to medicine. Rikki's superiors thought she was doing too many things at one time.

Rikki was so outraged that she went charging off to the heads of the department. She wore a blue dress, because she wanted a peaceful color, and she wanted to look proper. She was careful with her body language.

"I sat with my hands folded in my lap," she told Ron after her encounter with the chief of the OB-GYN department. "I didn't do any crossing of my arms on my chest. No sirree. Didn't want him to think I was closing him off. Could you imagine what would have happened if I came in with tight pants and leather boots. He would have thought I had a leather whip in my pocket."

Rikki explained her case at length. She told them about how her art was important to her. She said she didn't let it interfere with her role as a medical student. She explained that broad interests were good for a physician. No one disagreed with her. But they didn't change her evaluation either.

Two months later Rikki was back at Pennsylvania Hospital, taking the advanced Gynecology 300 course with her same detractors. She didn't change her behavior, but this time they gave her honors. To become familiar with Rikki was to love her.

□ □ □

Ron Cargill had probably traveled further culturally than any other American black in the class—from the ghetto street corners of Harlem and Camden, New Jersey, to the exclusive campus of the Penn medical school.

The ghetto that Ron knew wasn't just a poverty-stricken pocket in a city; it was a different world, a different way of life.

"When I'm in the ghetto," Ron told a white acquaintance, "I talk little, and the few times I do talk, I talk with a very angry look. You just hold yourself in a way to let everyone know that you're not somebody who is going to allow himself to be abused. Like in the ghetto somebody might try to feel me out and ask me for a quarter. I say 'nah.' But I don't just say it like 'nah.' I say it so everybody knows I'm not giving up nothing. And if anybody tries to take it from me, it's going to be to the death."

Even his unusual style of dress was part of the tactics he used.

"The hat says you're not average, that you're not to be confronted," he said. "You don't take liberties with a man wearing a hat like I wore. The hat allows me to be in seclusion, even with a lot of people around, because the brim covers my eyes. The hat and my overall attitude kept people from sitting around me. People stay away from you if you make them feel uncomfortable. And people felt uncomfortable with me and my hat."

Many socially and economically deprived people in this country are destroyed by the social system. Others become street wise and learn how to use it. Ron delighted in telling his white classmates how he discovered how to beat the academic system, something they had learned as children without ever knowing it.

Ron discovered in high school that anyone who got good marks could do just about anything he pleased. It was the only measurement that was depended upon and all unquantifiable virtues paled in comparison. Ron set about to boost his quantifiable measurements so he could have the freedom to do what he wanted elsewhere.

He was a bright student, so with a little application he was soon getting top marks at his high school in Camden. From there he went to Rutgers University in New Jersey, continued to do well, and went on to the sought-after Penn medical school.

By the time Ron reached Penn, he had mastered the techniques of surviving in academia just as well as he had developed his ghetto-survival tactics.

Some of the black students were joking about the proper care and feeding of teachers who could pass or fail them when Ron revealed some of his tactics.

"You don't treat a full professor the same way you treat an associate or assistant professor," Ron said, quietly taking control of the discussion. "You have to know who your attending is. You have to know how famous he is . . . the work he's done in the field.

"If you're taking something in his field, you better bone up on it to the max. If you don't, your evaluation is going to be bad. If you have something that is in conflict with what the full professor says, you bring it up humbly," Ron said, emphasizing "humbly" with a sweet tone in his voice.

"You don't just correct him. You say something like, 'I thought so and so,' or, 'Isn't there a paper that says such and such?' If you correct them in the wrong manner, you're in trouble."

Ron was apparently successful with his studies and his tactics because he impressed many of the physicians he worked under. As he became more secure, he abandoned some of his defenses. By the time the fourth year had arrived, he no longer wore his broad-brimmed hat to school.

But at the same time he became more separated from the black ghetto. Becoming disappointed with the changes of leadership among the Black Muslims and becoming more exclusively involved in medicine, he stopped traveling to the ghettos every weekend to spread the word.

And finally when the world-famous department of anesthesiology at Penn offered him a residency—a guarantee that Penn would put him at the top of their selections for Match Day—Ron made a drastic change in his career goal.

When asked about giving up plans to practice medicine in the black ghetto, Ron would say:

"I know I'm kind of slipping up on my obligations. But maybe after ten or fifteen years I'll get certified in medicine as well. You know a lot of anesthesiologists are certified in two specialties like anesthesiology and internal medicine. Maybe after I've done anesthesiology awhile I'll practice medicine outside the hospital."

Then, almost as though he was trying to save his original goal, in his mind at least, he would add, "Let's just say I'm submerging my obligations for a while by going into anesthesiology."

At the end of the 1960s, the Association of American Medical Colleges set a goal of increasing the proportion of minority students in medical school to 12 percent by 1975–76. When it did so, fewer than 3 percent of the students were black, mainland Puerto Rican, Chicano, or American Indian.

The number of minority students increased quickly, reaching a high of 10 percent of the first-year class in 1974. Some schools got the extra students by substantially lowering admission standards for minority students, a move that was challenged in the U.S. Supreme Court as discriminatory against whites.

Penn insisted that it never lowered its standards, but rather started a nationwide recruiting drive to attract the most gifted minority students in the United States.

Part of the campaign included hiring Iona H. Lyles, who spent all her time promoting minority student interests and traveling around the nation trying to attract gifted black students to Penn's medical school.

It would seem that Ms. Lyles and her program had been effective.

The average grade-point average (GPA) for a black student at Penn was 3.3, higher than the national average for whites and only 0.3 points below that of the average white Penn student. Nationally, the average minority medical student GPA was 2.7, which was 0.5 points below the white average and considerably below Penn's figure.

One of the complaints about the national program to increase the number of minority students was that many of these students failed to meet the challenge of medical school and that the attrition rate therefore was high. On a national level, 5 percent of minority students dropped out before the second year, compared to 1 percent for whites.

At Penn, only one minority student had failed to graduate since the affirmative-action program began a decade ago.

The national goal of boosting the proportion of first-year minority medical students to 12 percent by 1976 failed. By 1977 only 9 percent of the first-year students were from minority groups. The high cost of medical school and dwindling loan money were cited as major reasons.

35

The day hadn't even begun yet, but Jim Nestor was already worried about falling behind his self-imposed schedule.

"I'm going to have to be moving today," he said, glancing at the clock at the nurses' station. "I can see that already."

He had just come back from the clinical laboratories, where he had obtained the overnight lab figures on all of his patients.

It was only 7:45 in the morning. Rounds would not begin for another fifteen minutes. But Jim wanted to be ready for any questions his resident might ask him as they went from bed to bed, checking the progress of each patient.

Jim wasn't usually so rushed. At thirty-nine, he was the oldest member of the class of '78 and was probably one of the mellowest and least compulsive of them all. But no one could take Medicine 300 at the HUP and maintain peace of mind.

Medicine 300 was the most exhausting hospital rotation that the students took, and the HUP was the most demanding place to take it in.

Students in Medicine 300 had to work twelve-hour days, and they were on call every third night. This meant, essentially, that they worked most of the night and slept at the hospital.

As 8:00 A.M. approached, more students and physicians arrived, cheeks red and noses sniffling from the cold sunny morning. Most of the patients in nearby open rooms were already awake.

Many of them watched miniature television sets suspended near their faces by mechanical arms. They seemed oblivious to the growing noise from the nurses' station as people gathered to begin rounds. A newsboy went by, pushing a wagon filled with morning newspapers. A tall cart filled with plastic breakfast trays rattled down the hall.

Jim shook his head as he rushed to transfer the lab findings on patients from a scrap of paper to the charts at the nurses' station. The time for rounds was approaching quickly and he still had many numbers to write down.

He wanted to have the charts ready for Dr. William C. Groh, the twenty-eight-year-old resident who would lead the rounds and the physician to whom Jim was most directly responsible. Dr. Groh was an efficient, energetic physician who had a phenomenal and frequently used ability to quote research papers from medical journals.

At precisely two minutes before 8:00, Dr. Groh walked from the elevator in front of the nurses' station, hung up his coat, and almost immediately began the rounds.

Jim fell in line behind two others who had joined Dr. Groh and waited to recite the figures he had obtained. It would be a long day for Jim because it was his turn to be on call. He would be working for the next seventeen hours.

□ □ □

Match Day was only three days away and the students in the class of '78 were becoming increasingly nervous.

Most of the students would be staying near their telephones between 6:00 and 6:30 Tuesday night. Carol F. MacLaren, Penn's assistant dean for student affairs, had already sent out a notice saying that she would call unmatched students and give them the sad news at that time.

Instead of going to the lecture hall, where all of their classmates would receive notification of acceptance, these students would sit down in private rooms with their career advisers and discuss the options still available to them.

In the past, unmatched students got the bad news when they were with their luckier classmates, but medical educators found that this was inefficient, not to mention inhumane. Usually the unmatched students were in such a state of shock that they were not able to consider immediately what the next logical move should be.

Now they have all night to ponder their plight and all morning to plan a way out. By noon on Wednesday, they would know which of the available hospitals they would want to go to and would be ready to make contact with them as soon as it was permissible under the rules of the matching program.

The timing was so critical that the students' advisers would have the appropriate telephone numbers and hospital contacts before them, in writing, so that they could actually be dialing a number as the clock struck noon.

□ □ □

Rounds took less than an hour because Jim's team at the hospital—the A team, which included Dr. Groh and two first-year residents—had only thirteen patients. Sometimes the team would handle twice that number, but there had been many discharges for Team A recently.

One of the most difficult cases confronting the team this morning was that of Peggy Davete, a seventy-seven-year-old heart patient. During the night she had been transferred to the floor from the crowded medical intensive-care unit (MICU), which needed her bed for an emergency heart patient.

Since Mrs. Davete was clearly the sickest person being treated by the team, she had been put in a room with a window opening onto the nurses' station for easy observation.

She had a heart disease classification of four, which meant her cardiovascular system was so impaired that little could be done for her. She had less than a 10 percent chance of leaving the hospital alive.

"She doesn't look good," Dr. Groh said, bending down to the woman so that he could place his stethoscope on her chest. Immediately Jim and Dr. Donna Glover, one of the first-year residents, did likewise.

As the three hovered over her, Mrs. Davete paid no attention. She was barely conscious, struggling to breathe oxygen from the green plastic mask over her face.

"She knows the score," said Dr. Robert Kahn, a first-year resident who had been on call and had examined the woman during the night. "She has three brothers who died of MIs [myocardial infarctions, which are heart attacks]."

Dr. Groh put his hand on the woman's chest and felt her heartbeat beneath his touch. Dr. Kahn said something about electrocardiograms.

"Yeah, there was something on that in the *Annals*," Dr. Groh said, referring to the journal *Annals of Internal Medicine.* Dr. Groh discussed the research paper, finished his examination, and said that he wanted blood tests taken frequently in order to monitor her condition.

Led by Dr. Groh, Team A moved to the other patients. They went faster now because the pertinent information on these patients had been gathered and discussed during earlier visits.

The blood sugar of Mrs. Robinson, a seventy-four-year-old diabetic, had dropped to a disturbingly low level during the night, and Dr. Groh didn't like it. He ordered a reduction in the amount of insulin being administered and told Jim to take frequent blood samples to make sure that the sugar level did not rebound and go too high.

Another seventy-four-year-old woman, who had heart trouble and financial problems, was being released with prescriptions for drugs that she had no money to buy. It would be dangerous if she did not continue taking the drugs. Dr. Glover assured the woman that something would be worked out.

Moving rapidly down the hall to other rooms and other patients, Team A saw:

• A fifty-year-old anemic woman who was always tired and had a strange disorder that the doctors could not diagnose.

• A sixty-eight-year-old man who had senile dementia, diabetes, and probably a cirrhotic liver, the result of alcoholism, that would kill him.

• A fifty-five-year-old woman who was being referred to the surgeons because she needed a new heart valve.

• A sixty-nine-year-old woman who was waiting for tests to determine why her pancreas was inflamed.

• A forty-five-year-old man who might need a kidney transplant because medication was not helping him enough.

The team had two potential kidney transplant patients and would have a third before the day ended. One of the two already hospitalized was a seventeen-year-old youth who was refusing to take medicines.

"We're tissue-matching your family members so we can get the best kidney for you," Dr. Groh said to the sullen youth, who was wearing a jogging suit.

"We want you to be in good shape when you get the kidney, but you've got to take that medicine."

Lying in bed, the youth looked at Dr. Groh but said nothing. Just as Dr. Groh was explaining the importance of the drug, the phone rang. The boy picked it up and started a conversation as though Dr. Groh were not there.

Dr. Groh's portable call-monitor beeped. It was the medical admissions office. Three patients were being admitted and Team A was at the top of the rotation list for first choice. The medical department had five other similar teams in the hospital, and they took turns admitting new patients.

This was a significant responsibility. Team members spent hours examining each new patient and getting his or her medical history. The team also assumed all responsibility for the patient during his or her stay in the hospital.

The team at the top of the rotation for the admissions list took care in picking its patients, trying to select those who offered an interesting challenge and letting the other teams handle mundane cases that required a lot of routine, tedious work.

This time the admissions office had one patient with diabetes, another with severe bronchitis plus other problems, and a third with kidney trouble. Since Jim was on call with Dr. Groh and would be getting the medical history and doing the physical exam, Dr. Groh let him select the patient.

Jim chose the kidney patient—a twenty-year-old woman named Gloria Walters—because he wanted to learn more about kidney disease.

Half an hour later the admissions office called Dr. Groh again. This time it had two patients with diabetes and one with severe and long-standing diarrhea. Jim chose the diarrhea patient—a ninety-two-year-old man named Richard Henry Richardson.

Jim chose this patient because GI (gastrointestinal) problems were frequently encountered in emergency room medicine, a specialty that Jim was considering, and because the attending overseeing Team A this month was a GI specialist.

Every student knew that it was best to select patients with problems on which the attending physician was an expert because the resulting instruction was superior.

Richard Henry Richardson would not be an easy patient for Jim.

In fact, Jim would spend much of the afternoon and most of the evening with the elderly man.

Jim did not know whether he and his wife, Becky, would be spending the next several years in Philadelphia or in California; he had selected training hospitals in both places. He refused to tell anyone which hospitals he had ranked highest.

For obvious reasons, all students were secretive about their choices. Not only would it have been embarrassing if everyone knew that a student had not gotten his or her first choice, it also could put the student at a professional disadvantage. Would a hospital staff greet them with the same enthusiasm, students asked, if it were known that they had wanted to be at some other hospital but didn't make it?

Andrew Henderson already knew that he and his medical student wife would be going to Wilmington, and Suzanne Landis and Bill McKenna knew that they would be going to North Carolina. All of them had already been accepted by hospitals there.

This was permitted under the rules of the matching system. Since the heartless computer in Illinois could put one half of a couple in California and the other half in Massachusetts, hospitals were allowed to give special consideration to students who were married or even practically engaged.

It was also all right for Penn to guarantee Ron Cargill a spot in the anesthesiology program, so long as neither the hospital nor the student tried to use coercion by offering a match only if the other party promised to reciprocate.

Some students felt that the matching system was not completely honest and that many hospitals and students made deals with one another, which was not permitted.

It is difficult to prove this, but officials in Evanston said they had noticed a lot of "sham matching"—students listing only one hospital, presumably because they had been promised a spot or at least believed they had been promised one.

An average of 6 percent of the students in the matching program each year list only one choice. But many of these students apparently either misunderstand assurances from the hospital or are deceived, because in the end, 10 percent of them are not accepted.

Richard Henry Richardson was sitting in a chair near his bed, having considerable trouble opening the milk carton that came with his lunch because he had been partly paralyzed by a stroke. He greeted Jim with indifference, being more interested in his problems with the milk container than in Jim's questions.

It was a difficult interview and, with the physical examination, took almost two hours because the stroke had also left Mr. Richardson with expressive aphasia—that is, he could understand questions but had trouble in expressing his answers.

Mr. Richardson seemed remarkably healthy for someone his age. His reflexes were intact, with the exception of weakness on one side due to the stroke, and all of his organs seemed to be functioning adequately.

The only problem was that he had lost forty pounds recently and he had had diarrhea—though only at night—for three months.

Jim called the physician who had admitted Mr. Richardson to the hospital, but got little additional information. The physician said he did not know Mr. Richardson and merely happened to be working in the clinic when Richardson arrived. He said he admitted him because the old man became incontinent in the clinic and appeared to need a GI workup.

Dr. Groh was outraged when Jim told him about the Richardson case and what the other doctor had said. "He's using the hospital as a dumping ground," Dr. Groh said. "That's not right. This kind of patient will be in the hospital for the next four years."

It is not uncommon for nursing homes, relatives of elderly patients, and even some doctors to have such hard-to-care-for patients hospitalized and then to forget about them. They are sick enough to be troublesome to those around them, but they are not really sick enough to require hospital care. And with the cost of that care in places like Penn approaching $300 a day, such a practice was a vast waste of resources.

Dr. Groh, however, was not the sort of person to think long about things over which he had no control. Quickly becoming resigned to Mr. Richardson's presence, Dr. Groh told Jim what tests were needed to investigate the elderly man's weight loss and diarrhea and then left to check a third admission that Team A was getting, a transfer patient from the medical intensive-care unit.

Jim looked at the new watch he had just bought at Sears specifically for his Medicine 300 rotation. It was almost 5:00 P.M. He was far behind schedule. He had lost much too much time on the Richardson case. He still had to interview and examine the new patient with kidney disease, get blood samples from Mrs. Robinson and another patient, and run to the laboratory to get the most recent figures on Team A's patients.

"You lose five minutes here and five minutes there," Jim said, picking up the phone to call the laboratory. "But it adds up. Lose five minutes twelve times and you've lost an hour."

Television dramas suggest that hospital medicine consists of making brilliant diagnoses on the basis of subtle clues and saving lives with super drugs and modern technology. Actually, it is much more tedious than dramatic.

On a typical day, Jim spent most of his time tracking down information on the telephone, transcribing numbers from little pieces of paper to big pieces of paper, drawing blood from patients, and running back and forth to the laboratory with the blood samples or the results.

Only a few hours each day were spent in the intellectual excitement of discussing complex cases and weighing alternatives, which frequently would not substantially alter the course of the medical problem under scrutiny. The complexities and uncertainties of internal medicine drove some students to fields like surgery, where the action taken was usually definitive, if nothing else.

Jim had hoped to make up his lost time by being particularly efficient with the new kidney patient. If he was, he still might be able to get to the free staff dinner in the hospital cafeteria at 8:00, work up the MICU transfer patient, and get to bed at a reasonable time.

But it didn't work out that way. He lost five minutes while trying to find Dr. Groh to consult him on a matter involving kidney disease. The history-taking dragged on because the patient was drowsy from medication that the nurse had given her in accord with instructions from another physician. Another five minutes was lost to an electrocardiograph technician who kept losing her leads.

The new case was also more complex than Jim had expected and it took six pages of longhand to write up the history. Finally, he lost ten minutes talking on the telephone, trying to get the laboratory results on the blood samples he had brought up.

The lab had Mrs. Davete's results, but none for the diabetic Mrs. Robinson. It said it had not received Mrs. Robinson's blood.

Jim insisted that he had brought the sample up, but after he hung up, he began to fear that he had left it somewhere. He really didn't want to have to get another sample.

It was almost 9:00 P.M. by the time Jim got to the cafeteria, and all the good food was gone. Getting an extra scoop of ice cream in compensation and a couple of packages of crackers for the late-night grind, Jim sat down and ate what dinner there was.

□ □ □

Students worry much more than necessary about matching with a suitable hospital. Residents and attending physicians constantly tell them that, but it does no good. They still sweat out the last few days, wondering what they will be daydreaming about or dreading at this time next week.

Forty-three percent of the students in the class of '77 got their first choices and 85 percent got one of the top five hospitals they listed. Most students list ten hospitals, though the Evanston officials say that some match participants list more than 90 hospitals rather than leave anything to chance.

About five Penn students failed to match each year, Mrs. MacLaren said, but they inevitably found a hospital that would accept them before Match Day was over.

The officials in Evanston, of course, refused to give out specific information on the 1978 match results, which were known but not yet released. All they would say was that 13,376 persons had been matched and 1,978 had not. There were still 4,000 vacancies, more than enough, but perhaps not in the right specialty or right hospital.

Most of those who fail to get a match are graduates of foreign medical schools—both Americans and foreign-born students. In fact, the graduate of a foreign medical school is less likely to be matched than to make it— 1,021 foreign graduates matched compared to 1,054 who did not in 1978.

Only 6 percent of the graduates of United States schools failed to match. That still left 791 unmatched American graduates in 1978. Undoubtedly some of them were Penn students.

Just as Jim was completing his Medicine 300 rotation, the names of the successful and unsuccessful students were in certified mail pouches en route to medical schools throughout the country.

Eventually one of the pouches would reach Carol MacLaren's office. She would get the names of those who did not make it, and on Tuesday night she would give them a call.

□ □ □

Dr. Groh was waiting for Jim when he reached the nurses' station at 10:30.

"X-ray is having troubles with Richardson," Dr. Groh said the minute Jim got near him. "He's incontinent and they say they can't do the films. Will you go down there and straighten this thing out?"

It was night now and, almost as though on a schedule, Mr. Richardson was no longer able to control himself.

Jim would lose a lot more than five minutes on this one. And he still had to work up the MICU transfer.

Mr. Richardson, a thin little man with a mischievous manner, was sitting in a wheelchair in the middle of an empty hall when Jim arrived. He was glowering at the x-ray technician, who was at a nearby desk ignoring him by writing something on a piece of paper.

"She refuses to take my x-ray," he said, almost like a boy who was pouting over an injustice from an adult. "Take me back to my room."

"He's unstable," the technician said curtly. The odor of the instability was obvious, but Jim was able to prevail upon the technician to try to get the x-ray again.

Jim, the technician, and another assistant tried twice more to get the necessary films. Wearing a protective lead apron, Jim held the old man up in front of the x-ray machine. The man's legs were too weak to support him, and he was scared and couldn't stop shaking, no matter how much the technicians insisted.

Both attempts to get the pictures failed because of one technical problem or another. Finally, Jim gave up and wheeled the old man back to the floor.

Jim explained the failure to Dr. Groh, who just shook his head.

Then Jim got some more blood samples and went up to the clinical laboratories. He discovered Mrs. Robinson's missing blood, which had been found by another technician and was already analyzed.

Then he went down to the x-ray viewing room with Dr. Groh to look at some films of other patients.

The viewing room is an eerie place at any time, with the white glow of light panels for reading x-rays on all sides. But it's a particularly sinister place at night, when the spotlessly clean hallways of the seemingly deserted hospital are empty and quiet, and a lone radiologist sits before a lit-up film, dictating his observations to a machine as he nibbles on a bit of toast.

"What are our chances of getting a hit tonight?" Jim asked, meaning a new admission.

"Virtually zero," Dr. Groh said. The other teams were up for the next admissions.

Jim was relieved. It was almost 1:00 A.M. now.

"Forget the MICU transfer," Dr. Groh said as they reached the third-floor nurses' station again. "I worked him up already, so you can read what I wrote instead. It's late and it would be better not to wake him up now."

Jim spent ten minutes reading the report. Another shift of nurses had come in—the same shift that was going off duty when Jim started his long day seventeen hours earlier.

Things were fairly quiet now. Mrs. Davete was still in serious condition, but stable. Mrs. Walters, the young kidney patient, was in a deep sleep now, aided by the drugs she had been given. And old Mr. Richardson had finally dozed off.

Jim put the MICU transfer's chart back on the rack, got his coat, and said good night to the nurse.

It was 1:15 in the morning. He could get a few hours' sleep now in one of the student beds in the rehab building. But he'd be back in six hours, starting the cycle all over again.

The most disturbing thought of all for Jim was that this was what he had to look forward to all next year as a first-year resident.

Where? He didn't know. He'd find that out Wednesday.

36

Mark Reber was sitting in the garden courtyard of Children's Hospital, nibbling on a sandwich he had brought from home and pensively watching some children playing under the indoor trees.

He was preoccupied and uncomfortable with the thought that he would soon become a physician. The four years of education were almost completed, yet he did not feel he had learned enough to be legitimately considered a physician.

"I don't know as much, or think I am as skilled as I expected I would be by now," he said to a friend, sitting next to him on the bench. "I think my expectations were unrealistic."

Mark took a bite of the sandwich and reflected further. His friend said nothing because he knew that with Mark a pause in a conversation wasn't an invitation to jump in with something but merely indicated that Mark was composing the next thought he would eventually get around to expressing.

"I feel I am entitled to be called doctor," Mark said, finally continuing his train of thought but still looking at the playing children instead of his friend. "I'm entitled to that because I can see other people who aren't much more experienced who are called doctor. They have M.D. degrees and society recognizes them as doctors. So I am just as entitled. But I don't think I will be a doctor until I can really take care of people, and I can't do that yet."

The "300" courses, which were essentially junior internships, frightened Mark somewhat and made him more apprehensive about his impending postgraduate training as a first-year resident. He realized how hard he would have to work and the amount of responsibility that would be thrust upon him now, ready or not.

Mark's fears and concerns were not unusual—most of his classmates expressed similar feelings as the last of their medical school days ebbed away. And his concerns were not unrealistic either.

"When a medical student graduates," Dean Stemmler said, "he has a good general knowledge base and has good general skills to begin to provide direct care, but under supervision. He is not an independent practitioner. We don't view him as such and the law doesn't view him as such. He doesn't know how to care for patients without a lot of direction at this point."

Medical degree or not, Dean Stemmler saw the new graduate as essentially being only half of a physician. The first half of becoming a physician was the acquisition of information and technique. This was achieved in medical school. The second half of the transformation process was learning how to apply these things. The students would learn this as interns and residents.

"An internship is a difficult, intense work experience," Dean Stemmler said. "It's one of the hardest jobs in medicine. In a sense it's humiliating at a time when the student is growing in strength. Here, as a fourth-year student, he was at the top of the totem pole. Now he moves out into his internship and he's back at the bottom again. The student starts thinking that he is good and then he is put down again. It's a shakedown experience."

The students had a good idea of what to expect in the coming year and they certainly knew what they had just been through. So their last weeks in medical school were not particularly joyous.

The prevalent sense was one of anxiety over the future and some disappointment over the past. All of this was mixed with satisfaction and relief that at least medical school was all over. The four-year experience didn't significantly change the personalities of the students. The positive, socially concerned students weren't hardened or embittered by the four years. And, conversely, the cynical, selfishly motivated were not made idealistic.

Matt Lotysh was leaving medical school with the same sense of intense, almost conspicuous, sincerity he arrived with. Rikki Lights still had the same disregard for conventional standards and was still outraged by white male domination. Mark Reber was still sensitive and caring, and he was still a little intimidated by those who were not.

But like any intense learning experience, medical school still had significant impact on the students. If there was a common quality to the changes affected by the four years of medical education, it was probably toughening.

Many students said that they had become a little less open, somewhat more cynical, possibly even distant, in their professional if not their personal lives. But looking back on their four years, significantly different types of experiences stood out in the student's memories.

Since medical school rewarded knowledge more than empathy, Mark had worried about losing his own sensitivity.

"The fear is that you will become less sensitive," he said. "I had that fear, but I don't think it happened to me. If you don't have time to cultivate your sensitivity, you sort of lose it. By this I mean the sensitivity that you develop from art and literature and music. But then there is the other sensitivity that you have as a human being. I might have lost some of that first type of sensitivity, but I don't think medical school has affected the way I relate to people or my ability to be aware of their feelings.

"There have been times when I've seen patients treated badly by other people, times when I felt they had been brutalized. I felt a sense of outrage and complained to someone who I felt shared that outrage. But it's true that I rarely confronted the person who was treating the patient badly."

Mark felt it was possible for sensitive people to go through the brutalizing aspects of medical training without damage because there were enough sensitive people in the system from whom one could get support and reinforcement.

Mark had less blanket criticism for the medical system than he had before he entered medical school because he could understand more now why some things were the way they were. He could understand, for instance, why patients might be kept waiting or why an intern who had been on duty for twenty-four hours was brusque with a patient. Now when his nonmedical friends criticized doctors and medicine as a whole, Mark demanded that they be specific.

But he was still shocked by some of the business aspects of medicine where unnecessary surgery was done in profit-making hospitals owned by the doctors treating the patients. He resented the condescending attitudes some doctors had toward not only patients but nurses, clerical staff and orderlies.

"Doctors on the whole are a very self-impressed lot," he said. "Many of them earn a lot of money and feel themselves quite entitled to it. My feelings are that no one is entitled to it." He still didn't like the way the words "rich" and "doctor" went together.

□ □ □

Matt Lotysh wasn't so much apprehensive about his impending internship as he was anxious to get on with it. He explained to someone how he felt about medical school coming to an end.

"I feel completely empty and devoid of any excitement. All I want to do is to get into that goddamn operating room as an intern. I am ready to do it tomorrow. I am not enjoying all this free time now, having finished school and waiting to start the internship. It's not a time of my life when I want to sit back and rest on my laurels. I really want to go charging ahead. I have had enough of medical school. I don't want to take any more rotations. I am tired of the role of a medical student."

Like so many of his classmates, Matt felt medical school had helped him grow as a person.

"More than anything else, my personal growth has been ahead of my academic growth. And I came here as an academic cripple. I was really crass and crude and arrogant and cocky. Now I have a lot more personal security, so I don't have to resort to that approach anymore. Before I didn't have any academic security. I had always thought of myself as being a little dumb. I never had any reenforcement academically. I had always done physical things like selling insurance and diving for abalone. Now I've got it together both physically and academically. I am more happy about myself as a person right now than I am about having an M.D. after my name. The M.D. was something I had four or five years to become accustomed to. There was never any real doubt that I wouldn't get it. There was always a lot of doubt that I would ever get on the road to becoming the type of person I wanted to be."

Medical school had enabled Matt to see himself as being strong, capable, diligent in his desire to do his best, honest, caring of others, and certainly empathtic. "I don't think I would have scored myself high on any of these things when I came to Penn," he said.

It was difficult to say why medical school would give these things to Matt and a lot of other students, who expressed somewhat similar feelings of having found new self-worth. Undoubtedly part of it was the very difficulty of medical school. To master so much technical material, when at times the feat appeared impossible, couldn't help but give students a sense of self-worth and self-confidence.

The moment of mastery comes suddenly. A line is crossed and instantly the sense of competence outweighs the sense of ineptitude. Matt remembers how it happened to him:

"One day about a year ago I suddenly realized that I was a doctor. Literally over one afternoon's experience. I just decided I was a doctor. I had been waiting for this moment. It was almost orgasmic. I had a very strong feeling of warmth throughout my body. I felt very much in touch with my environment, very personally aroused, not in a sexual sense but an intellectual sense. I felt that my head and my body were really one and they were doing maximally what I had been trying to get them to do all these years. It was a sudden awareness . . . a sudden acquisition of confidence that I knew what I was doing."

The events leading up to the revelation sounded mundane in retrospect. He was on the GI service. He was rushed one afternoon and in a couple of hours had to admit three patients, getting their complete medical histories and doing careful physical exams. Then, without referring to notes, he made diagnoses and detailed the problems of all three patients to the attending on the service, a feat he thought impossible for him to do a year earlier. Under pressure he was able to do what a full-fledged physician would have had to do, and he did it well. At all times he was in charge of the situation. He had achieved mastery. He had become a physician.

□ □ □

Rikki Lights also made the discovery that she had become a physician, but she saw the same experience in a sharply different way. Both she and Matt were highly verbal people, capable of expressing themselves in a clear and vivid manner. But Rikki was an artist and her metamorphosis was seen in artistic terms.

All through medical school Rikki had been depressed and disheartened by her inability to find the art of medicine. All she seemed to be doing was collecting disconnected, dry facts that couldn't be manipulated by the creative process into a sum total greater than the parts.

It was a problem confronted by all medical students, who had to spend their first few years in school accumulating countless unfunctioning bits of knowledge—like the parts of a machine that had not yet been assembled.

Rikki's machine came together at the start of her fourth year. It, too, was a dramatic moment. Suddenly everything slipped into place and started working beautifully. Without realizing precisely what had happened, she had crossed the line that separated the acquisition of knowledge from the ability to apply it.

Rikki was working in the emergency room at the HUP when she realized that something was different.

"All of a sudden, one day, it went *Boom!*" she said, recalling the experience. "All of the knowledge I had sort of blossomed. Before, it was like a seed. But once I found out where I belonged emotionally, intellectually, and artistically in medicine, everything flowered.

"I really felt free to move about within the body of knowledge that we call medicine . . . to challenge it . . . to really question it and know that my questions were based upon astute observations . . . all of this happened in the emergency room. It was an awareness that I knew what I knew. I didn't have to go and ask for direction or advice. I began to trust myself. I realized that I knew a lot more than I thought I knew. How did it happen?

"My maturity and my knowledge and my own self-awareness increased to the point where all the things came together and I became a personality within the profession.

"The big thing I discovered was that medicine had a dialectic. It had an art of correct reasoning. I discovered the art to medicine."

After the revelation, Rikki began to take a delight in medicine and the faculty seemed to begin to take a delight in her and she began to get honors in one course after another. She was beginning to feel that she could create in medicine just as she had been creating as a writer. She finally knew enough to manipulate facts and find new truths.

Rikki's world of medicine intruded into her writing and probably always would now. Rikki went back to her old work and inserted characters who were sick. She wrote a poem—"Dissection"—which described her experience at the anatomy table during that first year. The first few lines read:

> I sat white-coated on a high wooden stool.
> Death fingers marked a trail faint as lace
> on nose tips sweating from body heat.
> We looked down with detached warm eyes—
> Our bodies alive,
> Our breath condensing into warm moisture
> melting the chill.
> Chests heaving in anticipation.
> Rubber-covered fingers wrapped firmly
> Around sharp scalpels.
> Waiting . . .

In addition to "Dissection," she had written a long poem about a suicidal patient whom she treated at Philadelphia General Hospital ("For She Who Wants to Kill Herself"), a poetic study of mental unbalance ("Origins of Fever"), and a piece about her life with Ron, medicine, music, and the stress that comes with a serious medical problem like her husband's ("Thunder Gates").

She began writing "A Is for Anatomy," a dictionary to familiarize children with the body. She reached "K Is for Kidney" on the day that the hospital called to say Ron would have to go on the kidney machine, and the experience was so shocking that she temporarily abandoned the work.

Ron's medical crisis began just after the start of school for Rikki. And as school ended, almost four years later, Ron still held on to life with the aid of the damnable machine.

"It's not easy," said Rikki. "It never was easy. It's certainly not getting any easier. If there's one thing I realize about renal failure, it's that it's unremitting. It runs rampant and there's very little you can do about it. I think Ron's remaining active does a lot to keep him stable. He exercises a lot. His body appears healthy, but there are just everyday things that go on with dialysis—nausea, weakness." The fistula the doctors wanted to replace was continuing to do well. They still wanted to give him another one, but Ron continued to refuse. "We don't want to be extravagant with Ron's flesh," Rikki said. "Ron's in good shape. We've got a lot to be thankful for. But renal disease is a progressive thing. Still, you don't have to let it dominate you.

"So you have renal failure. So you have cancer. So you have whatever. You don't have to let that be who you are. You don't have to define your life in terms of being a patient. And that's what we're trying to get away from.

"The big problem in our lives right now is the music industry."

Rikki laughed. She was right. It was difficult to make it in the world of music.

□ □ □

Like Matt Lotysh, Steve Levine found medical school valuable in helping him grow personally. He came to medical school tense, compulsive, and angry. He was still angry, but he was much calmer now and more secure in his command of life.

"Maybe someday I'll be able to say that I'm really glad I went to medical school because I'm a successful cardiologist who really loves his work. But right now I'm glad I went for a different reason," Steve said. "I'm glad for the personal growth experience that I have had. I'm much calmer, much more secure, much more self-confident, a hell of a lot surer of where I am. Just as the army was a big growth experience for me and college was a big growth experience so was medical school. Most traumatic experiences like that are important growth experiences."

Steve couldn't think of a single incident that profoundly affected him. It was more a mosaic of stressful experiences—autopsies, cadavers, difficult and bloody operations, the birth process, diseases that medicine was helpless to combat, watching people in pain and being unable to help, watching people die with the grief of their relatives all around, watching people die with no one around them to care.

Finding medical school less intellectually demanding than he had expected, Steve would leave Penn disappointed. The idealism of those in academia hadn't impressed him either.

"I have met some doctors who have a very idealistic approach to medicine. But most physicians in academia are fighting for grants. They are like the lawyers they hate. They argue. They fight. They're competitive. They're intellectual weight lifters. My grant can beat up your grant."

□ □ □

Constantly encountering such emotionally wrenching episodes as seeing people in pain or fear or near death has profoundly affected Jim Nestor, who also looked upon his medical education as a valuable experience for him as a person.

"It's inevitable in any one month that one of your patients is going to die," Jim said. "Say in one month you see forty people. One of them will probably die. Depending on the relationship you had with that person, the death can really bother you.

"I think one thing that medicine does for you is that it makes you very realistic about life and death and pain and what your body is all about. It takes you away from the glamorous television/movie picture scene and gives you a pretty heavy dose of reality. People don't see death anymore in America. Back in the old days when there were big families, death was a common part of life. You learned how to deal with it. People generally don't deal with death themselves anymore. They leave it to the nursing homes and doctors.

"By watching your own reaction to people dying I think that you learn a lot about yourself and a lot about how to help people get through it. People are scared when they're in the hospital. They're often in tight situations and you're there to sort of help them.

"You discover your own fears about death and pain when you help them. When people are obviously scared and obviously in pain you can't help but have some empathy for them. Part of it is just sitting back when it's all over and thinking about what your reactions were. Why was I angry? Why was I so upset? Why couldn't I go to sleep that night? That sort of thing. It might take a couple of weeks before you can sit down and think it through, but it's good when you do. You're forced into the situation where you really do have to think about what's going on in your world and inside your head."

Confronting death does make medical school a unique educational experience. Many students, however, deny that death affected them much. Faculty members believe that many of these students were denying things to themselves just as they escaped the stress of anatomy class with gallows humor.

But Steve Levine was concerned about it enough in the first semester to discuss his concerns openly with people, though he came to regret it because classmates put him down for it. Rikki Lights wrote about death. And Marge Shamonsky also mentioned it in reflecting on what medical school had meant to her.

She was particularly disturbed to discover how death was accepted with such indifference. It wasn't special at all. It was just part of the process.

"I used to think that if I was dying the whole world would be concerned. I certainly thought that my doctors would be concerned because they would have a personal interest in my death. But now I've seen what it's like in the hospital. I was so surprised to find out how matter-of-fact a thing death was. Someone in the hospital dies. Someone who might have been there for days or weeks. Someone whom everyone knew. And then they die. And they're dead. And it's over. Everything goes on as it had been going on before the person died. It's almost as if the death wasn't noticed by anyone but the person who died. I don't want to die in a hospital. I'd rather be at home, surrounded by people who cared about me."

Not everyone agreed that medical school had contributed to his personal growth. Speaking almost with anger, if not bitterness, Marge's husband, Randy Wiest, discussed his feelings about medical school:

"A lot of people change in medical school. But I think it's a change for the worse. They become less human. The medical meat grinder just makes them into the automotons you see in the HUP.

"Medicine has actually been a hinderance to my personal development. Apart from medical school, these four years have been remarkable. I fell in love, had my first serious relationship with a woman, got married, got into some intense interpersonal difficulties, really worked at the relationship, which seemed daily or every other week not to work. I feel I have grown as a person over the last four years, but medicine has been a hindering force. Having gone through a marriage relationship, I have a much better sense of who I am as a person. I'm really much more in touch with my feelings because of marriage than because of medical school.

"I'm kind of disillusioned. Medical school wasn't the quality-education experience that I thought it might be or that I thought it should be. It's really been a disappointment. I think it's such a low-yield experience. Much of the time you spend in clinical situations is wasted. You're just standing around and doing nothing, wasting a lot of psychic energy waiting for something to happen."

Was he sorry that he had gone to medical school?

"It's hard to say to yourself that you've just wasted four years of your life," he said. "What does that do to your self-image? I still have this underlying optimism of what I can do in medicine."

Randy was shocked by how far ahead students and physicians had to plan their lives.

"Isn't it incredible," he said, "that you start thinking of your life in chunks of time measured in years? Two years here, three years there. Before, it was all you could do to think about the next week or the next month. Now the big blocks of your life are beginning to look like a road map in front of you. It's kind of scary. The track has got to end someplace. You've got to get off the treadmill someplace. It's depressing to look ahead at your life and say I've got three years to do in a residency and two years to do in the Public Health Service and then maybe I can start living."

□ □ □

Some students feel that medical school has had some negative influences on their personal development.

Conrad K. King, Jr., said:

"I think it has made me a little less sensitive to certain things. I'm not as amenable to other people's problems. By other people I mean the people in my life—my family, my mother and father, my wife. I seem to have had medicine on my mind all the time, especially as it drew closer to the fourth year. I got more and more involved and had less of me for other people.

"It's made a different person out of me. I don't think I'm a worse person, just a different person. I guess I'm not the bubbly nice guy I thought I was when I first started. I guess maybe I'm a more serious person. Just seeing everything that we saw in those four years was . . . it was just sobering. It brings you down. Not so much death, just the fact that you have to take so much of yourself and put yourself into it to make the grade. You have to take the time and energy from other areas. Unfortunately the other areas are things like your socialization and things like dealing with your loved ones. You have to take it away from them."

Suzanne Landis said:

"I think I've become more cynical. I came to medical school having known only primary care physicians like my father and his friends. I never thought there was a thing like high-powered university medicine and this thing they call academia.

"I think that in a general sense, a very superficial sense, I am harder. I know one thing for certain. I used to smile all the time, even at people I didn't know. I used to converse with them. I find now sometimes I don't have the energy or the desire to converse superficially with acquaintances.

"I don't think any medical student can go through medical school and not become slightly cynical or hard. Not only do you see such abuses to patients, you see abuses to house officers. The abuses are passed down from the attendings to the fellows to the residents to the students and then perhaps to the patients. There are abuses to people in general."

Hagos Tekeste, from Ethiopia, felt medical school had discouraged him from showing as much emotion as he once did.

"For example," Hagos said, "if a patient dies I don't usually weep or show tears, whereas if I never came to medical school perhaps I would. It is part of the system. You are trained to be professional. I don't think there is anything wrong with being emotional. If anything, I think emotion should be encouraged to come out. The educational system does dampen emotional expression and I think that is bad. When you get together to review a case, you talk about manipulative things, like drugs, and not about the patient's emotions, not about your own emotions."

Richard Ellison doesn't feel medical school has changed his self-image, but it has changed the way he appears to other people.

"When I go home and see friends I have not seen before, they say 'Oh, doctor, oh doctor, you're going to be a doctor.' They seem to expect more from me than perhaps they did before."

Ron Cargill became less emotionally expressive, but he did not think it was a bad thing.

"It's part of medical training," he said. "You have an attitude, an atmosphere, about you. I say it's an attitude that commands respect. It's important. It serves a purpose. I think it's important to have a professional way about yourself, a professional attitude. It's part of the profession. I'm not going to speak against it. But I do maintain my ability to discard it."

Kate Treadway had one of the most positive things to say about medical school.

"It's hard to know beforehand how consuming medical school is going to be. That's not necessarily negative. It's fascinating. It's very seductive in the sense that at the beginning it was hard for me to stop thinking about medicine. I really had to make myself come to some sort of compromise with life outside of medicine. I guess I was surprised at how intensely someone could spend all of one's time thinking about medicine and being involved with it."

And so the students in the class of '78 reached the end of that process that turned laymen into physicians. In a few days they would be matched with their hospitals for postgraduate training and in a few weeks they would officially become doctors.

After going through the process with them, these students didn't look or act appreciably different from the way they did when they had come to Penn four years earlier.

Partly that was because knowing the process that turned them into physicians had stripped away much of the magic. The physician was no longer an all-knowing person who could speak authoritatively on all matters dealing with medicine. Rather he or she was a person who knew some things about medicine, but didn't know a lot about other things. It was deflating to realize that a specialized internist might know less about delivering a baby than a paramedic or maybe even a mother, for that matter. Or that a medical student could go through medical school without ever having witnessed a birth or ever having set a fractured limb. Or that a fireman might know more about resuscitating a heart attack victim than a dermatologist does.

Yet our society gives the medical profession the highest status. And if a patient doesn't look up to a trusted personal physician as a God, he certainly has imbued him with more wondrous abilities than the doctor could ever possibly achieve.

"One of the human attributes is always to attribute to the curer something that is mysterious or unknown," Dean Stemmler said. "I think that is because the patient wants to believe that there is something more than what we actually do know. The priestly role is an attributed role on the part of the population."

Dean Stemmler did not think that this was the result of the public's naïveté or ignorance. The public is quickly becoming much more sophisticated about such things. He said that even physicians who become sick imbue their personal physician with these special powers even though they should know better.

Steve Levine had similar things to say about this strange phenomenon of trust and elevation.

"Probably in every culture someone has to play the role of being an expert at dealing with disease," Steve said. "Whoever plays that role—whether it be shaman or midwife or doctor—is going to be imbued with special powers.

"Maybe we have taken some of the priestly and magical qualities out of it with modern medicine. Patients know that we don't invoke the gods or anything like that. We've taken the supernatural elements out of it, but we've replaced them with a technology that is so complex that it might as well be mystical because it is so far out of the reach of the average person's ability to comprehend or to control it himself.

"Maybe in the old days it was only the priest who knew how to call in the right gods. Now the physician is the only one who knows how to analyze the situation and plug in the right machine. Pain and death are so fearful that people have to invest those in charge with special powers.

"There's an emotional payoff in believing in your doctor. You go to your doctor about this pain that won't go away and you don't know why it's there. It's getting worse and it's been going on for several days. You think of cancer and you think of early death. You've gone through all this alone and the thoughts get worse as you're sitting in the waiting room wondering what it is and what can be done about it. Considering all this, it's a little comforting to think, as you are being ushered into your doctor's office, that, whatever it is, he will be able to take care of it."

37

After four years of work, it was finally Match Day. The students didn't start drifting into Lecture Room A until a few minutes before noon.

It was the same lecture hall in which the students had gathered for the first time as a group four years earlier to be welcomed to the medical school. The mood in Lecture Room A was, however, much more festive this time.

A couple of students had brought in small bottles of liquor to toast the occasion. Walter Tsou was standing at the bottom of the amphitheater lecture hall with a camera, taking pictures of his classmates.

Barbara Turner was all smiles. She had just returned from a five-week vacation in England. Rikki Lights was sitting alone in the tiered amphitheater, her legs hunched up under her chin, staring down into the speaker's pit.

The rumor spread through the group of students that there was going to be a surprise announcement. Something very exciting had happened to one of the students in the class. The students looked around at one another, wondering what it could be.

Kate Treadway was there with her husband and four-month-old baby, Michael. With characteristic care in the planning of her life, Kate had given birth in November, just after she had completed her courses, so she would have ample time to be with Michael before starting her internship in June.

Many students hadn't come to Lecture Room A this day.

Once again Helene Silverblatt was in Peru with her sister and the natives of the small village of Sarhua. She had applied for a residency in psychiatry. Her unusual ability to relate to people would be put to good use in such a specialty.

Jim hadn't come to Lecture Room A either. He had heard that in prior years disappointed students had broken down and cried or appeared to be in obvious pain. He didn't want to see this happen to people he had become fond of over the last four years. So instead he did some shopping, got his car fixed, and made plans to call Carol MacLaren at 2:00 P.M.

Matt Lotysh was not there either. He was in California with his seventy-one-year-old father, who had developed rectal cancer. Matt had made the diagnosis himself.

He happened to be home, preparing for interviews at California hospitals, when his father told him he had been feeling bad lately. He had lost weight. And his bowel habits had changed.

Matt did an examination. He felt a mass in the rectum. His father's liver felt bumpy. Matt's father had all the signs of rectal cancer, but this time Matt hoped his diagnosis was wrong. It wasn't.

"Congratulations to all of you. I'm sure you thought this day would never come."

It was the voice of Carol MacLaren, yelling up from the speaker's pit. Standing with her were three other people, holding stacks of envelopes in their arms.

Mrs. MacLaren explained that they would distribute the envelopes, each one addressed to a different student. The envelope contained the name of the hospital the student had been matched to. It wasn't a letter, but rather only a computer print-out on a slip of paper. It said merely that student so-and-so had been matched with hospital program such-and-such.

Finishing the brief explanation, Mrs. MacLaren invited the students to get their envelopes, and the rush was on.

In a group, the 142 students in the room rushed down to the people distributing the envelopes in alphabetical order.

Some of the students ripped open their envelopes as soon as they got their hands on them. Others took their envelopes and found a private corner or ran out into the hall to look at the results by themselves.

Rikki Lights looked stunned after reading her match.

"How did you do?" she was asked.

"Huh, okay."

"You look shocked," someone else said.

"It's anticlimactic," she said. "It's the end of freedom. I'm sad because, wow, this is it. This is official medicine from now on in."

Rikki had been matched with Presbyterian Hospital in Philadelphia.

The big news involved Katharine Treadway. She had been matched with Massachusetts General Hospital in Boston, the best, most prestigious, most sought-after hospital of them all. No one else in the class achieved this. Kate seemed subdued, but obviously happy. She and her husband kissed and drank a toast from a small flask they had brought with them.

Mark Reber also got his first choice—St. Christopher's Hospital in Philadelphia. Mark chose St. Christopher's because he thought that the program was less academically high-pressured and oriented more toward community medicine than Children's Hospital, Philadelphia's only other pediatric hospital and Mark's second choice. "Now we can start looking at real estate ads," he said.

Mark called his wife, Karen, and told her that he had been matched to a hospital in Philadelphia. Karen sighed with relief. A native New Yorker, she had come to like Philadelphia and didn't want to leave.

Jim's wife, Becky, wasn't so lucky. Her husband had been matched with the Kaiser Foundation in Santa Clara, California.

No one cried openly but one student was close to tears as he pleaded with Mrs. MacLaren to find out what he could do now. He had matched, but way down on his list of choices, and now he didn't want to go.

Only one of the 142 Penn students who got the results this day didn't match. Precisely at noon—in accordance with the rules—this student's adviser started calling hospitals around the country to see if any had openings that his student might fill.

By 2:00 P.M. they had found a spot for him in a university hospital in a midwestern city.

All told, 52 percent of the Penn students were matched with their first-choice hospitals. Eleven percent got their second choice and 10 percent their third. Eighty-three percent got one of the top four choices.

Richard Ellison got a psychiatry residency at the New York University Medical Center.

Conrad King would take medicine at Bryn Mawr Hospital, an affluent community hospital just outside Philadelphia.

Steve Levine would take medicine at the University of California Hospital in Los Angeles. Matt Lotysh would also go there on a surgical rotation.

Helene got a pyschiatry residency at the Bernalillo County Medical Center, which was connected with the University of New Mexico.

Deborah Spitz would study psychiatry at the University of Chicago Hospital and Clinics.

Hagos Tekeste would go to Presbyterian Hospital with Rikki, where he would study medicine. Walter Tsou would be there in the medicine department also.

Barbara Turner got one of the sought-after spots in the department of medicine at the HUP.

And Randy Wiest would escape the confines of an eastern city for the scenic splendor of Denver, where he would study family practice medicine at Mercy Hospital.

□ □ □

Within a half hour after they had arrived, the students in the class of '78 were gone, and once more Lecture Room A was empty.

For the students it was a supremely important moment, but the process of giving out the information happened so fast that it was almost as though it had never taken place.

There were no lunch celebrations by large segments of the class. No big gala took place in the Macke room. The students just vanished after they got their computer print-outs.

Outside on Hamilton Walk were only a few undergraduates. And every now and then a white-coated physician would hurry by on his way to or from the nearby HUP. It was a sunny day. Spring was in the air. But the trees were still bare. Nature's eternal cycle from winter to spring was not yet obvious.

The students wouldn't graduate from medical school for another two months and it wouldn't be until a month after that that they started their work as interns or first-year residents at the hospitals.

A few of the more compulsive students would use some of the time to take a couple of extra courses in areas they felt uncomfortable in, the thought being that they might learn one little additional thing that would make a big difference in the outcome of treatment for one of their patients. But most of the students would rest before starting the big push as brand-new physicians.

The three months would be filled with a mixture of satisfaction for having completed school and apprehension over beginning the next and final phase of their educational process. But the most strongly felt emotion would be a growing sense of excitement. Any move is exciting for people at this stage of their life and careers. But it would be especially exciting for these graduates because not only would most of them be moving to new cities, but they would be moving there as physicians.

Like it or not—and most of them liked it—they would be treated specially now. Everywhere they went they would be addressed as "Doctor."

In the street, at parties, in restaurants, people would treat them with some deference. As a group, they might come under repeated attack for their high incomes, and the high cost of medical care, and for not making house calls, and for the impersonal nature of modern medicine. But as individual physicians, they would be looked up to now, especially by their patients, who would have a vested interest to believe in them.

INDEX

women students (*continued*)
   lack of role models for, 119, 222
   men students and, 65–70
   patients' attitudes toward, 215–17
   percentage of, 128
   residencies for, 222–23

   sexism encountered by, 215–20, 221

Zinbar, Robert, 118, 121, 123–24, 125–26
Ziobrowski, Dr. Thomas, 131